Public Health Informatics

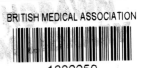

Public Health Informatics

Public Health Informatics
Designing for Change—A Developing Country Perspective

Sundeep Sahay
Professor, Department of Informatics University of
Oslo, Norway

T. Sundararaman
Professor, School of Health Systems Studies, Tata Institute
of Social Sciences, Mumbai, India

Jørn Braa
Professor, Department of Informatics University
of Oslo, Norway

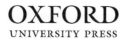
OXFORD
UNIVERSITY PRESS

OXFORD
UNIVERSITY PRESS

Great Clarendon Street, Oxford, OX2 6DP,
United Kingdom

Oxford University Press is a department of the University of Oxford.
It furthers the University's objective of excellence in research, scholarship,
and education by publishing worldwide. Oxford is a registered trade mark of
Oxford University Press in the UK and in certain other countries

Published in the United States of America by Oxford University Press
198 Madison Avenue, New York, NY 10016, United States of America

British Library Cataloguing in Publication Data

Data available

Library of Congress Control Number: 2016951476

ISBN 978–0–19–875877–8

Printed and bound in Great Britain by

Ashford Colour Press Ltd

Foreword

While human capacity to digest large numbers of statistics, and to translate those statistics into public health action, may have increased only piecemeal, the demand for data and statistics is expanding exponentially. The 2030 Agenda for Sustainable Development, with 17 goals and 169 targets, illustrates this increasing demand. Well over 200 indicators have been proposed for global monitoring of the Sustainable Development Goals, and for virtually all indicators disaggregation by all relevant stratifiers are considered essential. In addition, there is much emphasis on local analysis and use of data for decision-making.

On the supply side, innovations in technology and greater affordability of digital devices have created much excitement and action in the world of data. The highest echelons in government are speaking about a data revolution. Many hope that the data revolution will allow low and middle-income countries to leapfrog many development obstacles.

Health is no exception. There is much demand for 'real time' data for decision-making. Such data not only include disease surveillance, but also performance of the health services, administrative data, and population health monitoring, including risk factors and determinants outside of the health sector. In healthcare, local disaggregated data collection, analysis, and communication are additional priorities, directly linked to programme implementation and priority setting.

The opportunities to introduce and use individual electronic health records, interoperable databases, geospatial databases, web-based platforms, and SMS-based platforms for reporting health facility data, data warehouses, and so on have been seized by many countries' projects and researchers. The benefits for public health have, however, been modest compared to the levels of excitement and investment.

This book by Sahay, Sundararaman, and Braa helps us understand why these benefits have fallen short of our expectations and provides clear guidance on the way forward, with a focus on low and middle-income countries. They challenge the concept that public health informatics is a subdiscipline of health informatics, and turn this idea on its head. Using an array of empirical examples from many parts of the world, the authors build a convincing case for a broad definition of (expanded) public health informatics as the discipline that should encompass clinical informatics, electronic medical records, big data, and so on.

The arguments are built up from the perspective of information demand and population needs. While innovation and technology are critical drivers of the data revolution, they are often not sufficient as a solution. Furthermore, the effective use of information technology requires a thorough understanding of the national health information systems in low and middle-income countries. All three authors have been working for decades in field of information technology for health, which is evident through their arguments, examples, and proposals that enrich this book. Most notably, they have been the global driving force behind a web-based platform for health facility data reporting (and local analysis and feedback), which has become a remarkable success in many low and middle-income countries. The secret behind this success is not only the improvements in information technology, or the authors' remarkable persistence in developing the web-based platform with strong involvement from country stakeholders, but the simple fact that its development was fully grounded in public health needs.

The public health data gaps in low and middle-income countries are well known. Inadequate data for public health action are due to major data gaps, quality problems, timeliness issues, including public health emergencies, and poor dissemination and use. Inadequate data affect individual healthcare, quality, and safety due to poor paper-based and fragmented electronic systems. There is a lack of knowledge about major public health issues because of gaps in knowledge about human behaviour, environmental issues, biomedical aspects, and so on. And many countries are not able to monitor progress to major international, regional, and national targets, such as the health-related Sustainable Development Goals.

The field of public health informatics, in its expanded version as proposed in this book, has much to offer to address these deficiencies in the coming years. Effective linkages will have to be ensured with strengthening health statistical capacity, both technical and institutional; new non-traditional sources of data and metadata, including big data, need to be leveraged; open data should be promoted—that is, open access to data respectful of national and international data policies, promoting transparency and ensuring accountability; new and effective public and private collaborations need to emerge. Above all, this requires a holistic approach that brings together multiple producers and users, considering multiple uses with a focus on population health, and all kinds of data—including clinical, population, and spatial—which are all nicely captured here by the term public health informatics.

Ties Boerma, MD, PhD
Director, Information, Evidence, and Research
World Health Organization
Geneva, Switzerland

The Independent Expert Advisory Group (IEAG) on a data revolution for sustainable development: http://www.undatarevolution.org/wp-content/uploads/2014/11/A-World-That-Counts.pdf

Preface

This book is the chronicle of a struggle—a quiet, intense, and prolonged engagement by a remarkably diverse community of practitioners and academics to address one of the most unexpectedly intractable problems of modern public health. There was an age of innocence in the opening days of the engagement in the 1980s, when the narrative was of a malfunctioning public health system in low and middle-income countries (LMICs), which would be set right through modernization using information and communications technologies (ICTs). The expectations of ICT cannot be faulted, and in sectors such as banking and transport, ICTs have indeed helped to revolutionize performance. But as project after project in public health fails to live up to these expectations, and cycles of innovation to obsolescence become shorter and shorter, there is an air of bewilderment among health systems managers and administrators, and of denial combined with a stubborn techno-optimism amongst the technologists that the next wave of ICTs will fare better. However, the results show we are often barking up the wrong tree, trying to find solutions for wrong problems.

Despite all the problems and travails, public health informatics is today more recognized as an integral and essential part of any health systems strengthening or reform effort than it was two decades back. With this difference—that it is no longer an unqualified tool, or a subject of the reform process but equally an object of reform. Health information systems are now better portrayed as co-evolving with health systems—requiring similar policy environments for facilitation, overcoming institutional barriers, and responding similarly to political choices (with regard to power and equity) in the design of systems.

However, this rather negative portrayal of problems that beset current public health informatics should not in any way detract from the potential it has to revolutionize the performance of healthcare systems in LMICs, or the need to do so, or the determination to work towards this end. Gramsci's motto expresses the spirit of our enterprise best: 'Pessimism of the intellect, optimism of the will'. It is the duty of academic thought to lay out the problems, barriers, and approaches, just as it is the task of implementers and governments to factor these in and move forward, without recreating the same mistakes.

This book is addressed to the domains of the academician, the practitioner/ activist, and the policy maker. It is meant to help them reflect on their own experiences, help understand the roots of some of the 'wicked' problems experienced, and to plan work ahead. Most practitioners—whether they are providers or users of information, or IT managers and developers—have implicit programme theories of how ICT would improve health sector performance, and these narratives can often be contradictory. This book highlights many such understandings and tries to make practitioners' tacit knowledge more explicit not only to themselves, but also helps them understand the same problem through the eyes of the 'other'. To the academician, we hope this book will help theorize and research a number of domains that have not drawn appropriate academic attention because they are seen as operational issues, or because it has been so difficult to adopt multidisciplinary approaches. To the policy maker, this book will help in the transition in thinking from 'good policy, poorly implemented' to a 'policy that is only as good as it is implemented'. This is also about persuading the leaders to acknowledge that underperformance of health information systems cannot be dumbed down to simplistic understandings of 'garbage in, garbage out', but arise from fundamental problems of design that policy makers are, at least in part, accountable for.

This book is written at a juncture when the new discipline of public health informatics is just emerging, and its scope and boundaries are still fuzzy and in the making. This emergence has many drivers some of which are seeing similar exponential growth across all geographic and social contexts. These include changing informational needs, emerging technological platforms, and new global health reform agendas—all of which are forcing us to radically revise and rethink public health information systems and its foundational conceptual premises. But at the same time there are other dimensions like institutional capacity, socio-cultural systems, or the maturity of health systems, in which change is much slower and deeply context specific, and the discipline is challenged to elucidate lessons that are more universal. But one of the central themes of this book is that this fuzzy, embryonic character of the enterprise allows us scope to define this discipline in a much more expanded, flexible, and open-ended manner than many of the pre-existing definitions.

This book is written by a team who can describe themselves equally as academicians, activists, practitioners and, to some extent, also as involved in policy-making. This book is therefore a chronicle of our respective personal and collective struggles over the last decade and a half (at least) to materialize the potential that ICT promises towards designing a more effective public health system that is also more decentralized and participatory. The contents of this book, in terms of the examples we choose, are lessons that we have drawn which are shaped by this shared and yet very diverse range of experiences from a multiplicity of contexts.

Two of the authors, Sundeep Sahay and Jorn Braa, are initiators and developers of the 'Health Information Systems Programme (HISP)', an innovative global programme of the University of Oslo initiated in the mid-1990s, designed to develop capacities in LMICs on public health informatics. Central to HISP is the development of a product called DHIS, or the District Health Information Software, on which work began in South Africa in 1997 as part of the effort to build a new and equitable healthcare system in the newly liberated nation. It continues to be inspired by the principles of heath IT systems that are open source, collaborative, and developed in a not-for-profit environment—and of health systems which are decentralized, district-based, and pro-poor. Today over 55 nations across Africa, Asia, and Latin America use DHIS 2 as one of their main products—and many of them operate, develop, and grow without reference to the initiating institution of HISP. The third author, Sundararaman's engagement began in 2007 as the Executive Head of the National Health Systems Resource Centre, India's apex technical support institution for the National Rural Health Mission (NRHM). A key facet of this role was to shape the development of public health informatics to support the NRHM's mission of strengthening decentralization, integration, and evidence-based decision-making in India. He has also been working on policy issues related to health systems strengthening and health equity over two decades as part of health rights advocacy with the People's Health Movement. He currently teaches at the School of Health Systems Studies, in the Tata Institute of Social Sciences in Mumbai, India. From 2005 onwards, the three authors, collaborating in academics, practice, and policy, have shared the warm appreciation that significant advances brought, but more often consoling themselves at all the near misses—the what-could-have-been scenarios—and still moving ahead, trying to shape the future while learning from the past.

But this book does not only represent the personal experiences and learnings of the three authors, but also represents the contributions from a large number of our colleagues and students—some of it during structured workshops, but a lot of it while interacting on the job, including doctoral thesis work. In particular, we acknowledge the benefits we have had from the rich discussions with Dr Arthur Heywood, independent consultant and one of the founding members of HISP in South Africa, affiliated to the University of Oslo and now stationed in Tanzania and his wide-span African experience in implementing health information systems. In addition, a notable mention should be made of Bob Joliffe, the reclusive Irishman who is also our pre-eminent advisor on the political economy of standards and all things ICT, and of Prof Geoff Walsham, University of Cambridge, who has urged us to ask the question 'Are ICTs helping to create a better world for us to live in?' Many of our case studies have been based on oral or written contributions from our colleagues, friends, and multiple doctoral students at the University of Oslo, and we would like to thank them also. We also acknowledge the learnings and shared experiences from the International Seminar on Public Health Information Systems that was organized in October 2014 at Chennai, by the Center for Technology and Policy, IIT Madras, and HISP India, which have stimulated us and contributed to the writing of this book.

We also note that though many of the case studies are critical of design and outcomes, this should not diminish the efforts that went into shaping them and the major technical achievements and learnings that some of them represent. Many of these case studies have since learnt from their own experience and moved on—but we capture them at a point of time, to be used as a learning tool, and to plan better for the future—across research, practice, and policy.

Putting together this book has been a long and creative process. At the end of it, we do not offer a simple list of solutions or recommendations. What we offer is a somewhat hypothetical, tentative, exploratory, and critical discussion on some key principles of design, clubbed together as 'designing for change'. This we hope will help and guide us on how to move forward incrementally towards realizing the truly immense potential of public health informatics to transform the health of populations across all nations.

Sundeep Sahay, Oslo, August 2016
T. Sundararaman, Mumbai, August 2016
Jorn Braa, Oslo, August 2016

Contents

Abbreviations

AaaS	Analytics as a Service		HIE	health information exchange
AAMRL	American Association of Medical Record Librarians		HIPAA	Health Insurance Portability and Accountability Act
AEHIN	Asia E-Health Information Network		HIS	health information system
			HISP	Health Information Systems Programme
AHIMA	American Health Information Management Association		HITECH	Health Information Technology for Economic and Clinical Health
ANC	antenatal care			
ANM	auxiliary nurse midwife		HIV	Human Immunodeficiency Virus
ANT	Actor–Network Theory			
API	application programming interface		HMIS	health management information system
ART	antiretroviral therapy		HMN	Health Metrics Network
CCG	Clinical Commissioning Groups		HWR	health worker registry
CDC	Centers for Disease Control and Prevention		IaaS	Infrastructure as a Service
			IAD	Institutional Analysis and Development
CDSS	clinical decision support system		ICD	International Classification of Diseases
CHE	catastrophic health expenditures		ICT	information and communications technology
CR	client registry			
CRVS	civil registration and vital statistics		IDSP	Integrated Disease Surveillance Programme
CT	computed tomography		IDSR	Integrated Disease Surveillance and Response
DANIDA	Danish International Development Agency		IP	internet protocol
DFID	Department for International Development		IPD	inpatient department
			IS	information system
DHIS	District Health Information Software		ISMR	Institutional Service Monitoring Report
DHIMS	District Health Information Management System		ISO	International Organization for Standardization
DHMT	district health management team		IT	information technology
EHR	electronic health record		LIS	laboratory information systems
EMR	electronic medical record		LMIC	low and middle-income countries
EPI	Expanded Programme on Immunization		LMIS	logistic management information system
FOSS	free and open source software			

M&E	monitoring and evaluation	PHC	primary healthcare
MoH	Ministry of Health	PHE	Public Health England
MCTS	Mother and Child Tracking System	PHI	public health informatics
MDG	Millennium Development Goals	PICMS	Pregnancy and Infant Cohort Monitoring System
NGO	non-governmental organization	PEPFAR	US President's Emergency Plan for AIDS Relief
NHIN	National Health Information Network	RBF	result-based financing
		RHIE	Rwanda Health Information Exchange
NHS	National Health Service	RIMS	Routine Immunization Management System
NHSRC	National Health Systems Resource Centre	RIS	radiology information system
NORAD	Norwegian Agency for Development Cooperation	SaaS	Software as a Service
NRHM	National Rural Health Mission	SARS	Severe Acute Respiratory Syndrome
NIST	National Institute of Standards and Technology	SDG	Sustainable Development Goals
OpenHIE	Open Health Information Exchange	SHR	shared health record
		SLA	service level agreements
OpenMRS	Open Medical Record System	SSH	secure socket shell
OMR	optical marker reader	SSHD	solid state hybrid drive
OOPE	out-of-pocket expenditure	TB	tuberculosis
OPD	outpatient department	TS	terminology service
OpenHIE	Open Health Information Exchange	UHC	universal health coverage
		UK	United Kingdom
OpenMRS	Open Medical Record System	US	United States (of America)
PaaS	Platform as a Service	USAID	United States Agency for International Development
PACS	picture archiving and communication system	WHO	World Health Organization
PBHR	personal-based health record	WTO	World Trade Organization
PC	personal computer		

Chapter 1

Public Health Informatics: Positioning Within an Informatics Framework

1.1 Public Health Within an Informatics Framework

This chapter aims to articulate public health informatics (PHI) within a primarily informatics framework. This feeds into Chapter 2, which situates PHI within a primarily public health perspective, enabling the development of a more holistic conceptualization on PHI. This chapter sketches out the landscape of PHI situated within the larger context of health and medical informatics as well as informatics for primary healthcare, which taken together, help to define the scope of this domain.

As a first step, we discuss within a historical perspective the broader discipline of informatics, or information systems, as it is often popularly called. This brief historical tracking helps to understand how the primary influence on health informatics has been the field of informatics and its application to business, rather than from a strong public health perspective. Next we position PHI semantically and conceptually among informatics in general: health informatics, medical informatics, and bioinformatics, in particular. This helps to elucidate on what is the distinctive focus of PHI, what this domain covers, and how different health information systems (HIS) relate to, but are not in themselves descriptive of PHI.

1.2 Our Point of Departure

To make clear our point of departure, we take the analogy of the computer and the human body, and relate those to the disciplines of computer science and health informatics, respectively. Computer science is concerned with the study of 'computers and computing', going into the nitty gritty details of the computer, programming languages, the algorithms underlying the programs, and other supporting hardware and software. In contrast to computer science, the discipline of 'information systems' examines the relationship between computer systems and organizations, teams, societies, and nations, basically trying to understand the different facets necessary to 'make information systems to work effectively'. So, the concern is not only if the computer is technically efficient, but also how it is 'organizationally implemented' and can bring value to institutional and human processes. This focus does not of course preclude the understanding of individual computers and applications, but that is just a matter of granularity of the focus. Information systems is thus about understanding the phenomenon from the level of individual machines and the people who use them, through to the different levels of granularity of teams, departments, organizations, nations, societies, and the global context.

Analogous to the above is the field of health informatics, which focuses on the individual patient and the internal workings of the human body, similar to how computer science focuses on the inner workings of the computer. The focus is on understanding these internal workings through applying information technology (IT) to health, manifested through clinical support systems, electronic medical records (EMRs), radiology informatics, and various others. The field of PHI is fundamentally about populations, and in studying that, is concerned about different levels of granularity from the individual patient, to health programmes, the health sector, ministry, communities, and entire populations. PHI is thus similar to the discipline of information systems, focused on understanding how IT is applied to the study of health in different levels of collectives that comprise the population. PHI is situated with information systems in the understanding of how IT can help in bringing improvements to public health. This foregrounds the need to understand issues of coverage, denominators, and indicators, which can be analysed at different levels of granularity. More importantly, PHI, because of its grounding also in informatics, can represent understandings of how to build effective systems, something which medical practitioners promoting health informatics do not necessarily prioritize.

In this chapter, we argue that health informatics as an academic discipline has focused primarily on the individual patient, and this has constrained thinking about the broader situation of the health of populations. This need not be the case, for if we seek to develop scalable design principles, we can seamlessly transcend different levels of granularity from the individual to the whole population. The focus on one does not preclude the understanding of the other, and the levels in between. This chapter then seeks to formulate these design principles which underlie the study of PHIs in low and middle-income countries (LMICs).

1.3 A Historical Overview of Developments in Computer Science and Informatics

1.3.1 A note on terminology

We begin with a small note on terminology. There are various terms to describe computer-based developments and their applications, including computer science, IT, informatics, and information systems. Also, in contemporary parlance there are new terms prefixed with the letter 'e'. Analogously, the terms used on the health domain include HIS, health informatics, e-health, and others. Very broadly, the term 'information systems' comes from North America, and seeks to understand the relation between computer-based systems and organizations. The inclusion of the term 'systems' reflects an expansion of the concerns from just the technical systems, to issues of organizations, people, culture, and various others.

In 1957 the German computer scientist *Karl Steinbuch* coined the word '*Informatik*' by publishing a paper called *Informatik: Automatische Informationsverarbeitung* ('Informatics: Automatic Information Processing'). The German word *Informatik* is usually translated to English as '*computer science*'. Primarily, *Informatics* or *Informatique* (as used by the French) is of European origins. A Russian scientist (A.I. Mikhailov) from Moscow State University was also one of the early users of the terms *Informatik* and *Informatikii*. In a book published in 1976, he defined informatics as the science that 'studies the structure and general properties of scientific information and the laws of all processes of scientific communication' (Nelson and Staggers 2013). From the 1960s, the word *Informatique* began to appear widely in the French literature and also in German as *Informatik*. In Norway, Kristin Nygard was instrumental in establishing the Institut for Informatik at the University of Oslo in the mid-1970s that had as its focus not only computing, but also systems design and development and their implementation in workplace settings. In the United States and the United Kingdom, the term informatics was not generally used. However, the term medical or health informatics began to appear in English publications in the early 1970s, and 'health informatics' represents a North American and UK usage of the term of informatics, primarily by clinicians and medical practitioners, in a technical sense of applying computers to patient-level health.

In this book, we have consciously adopted the terminology of 'public health informatics' (PHI) based on more than 20 years of research and practice within the Health Information Systems Programme (HISP), a research and development organizational network loosely coordinated by the Department of Informatics, University of Oslo. PHI includes aspects of technology—hardware, software, networks, systems development methodologies, and techniques such as prototyping, and their applications in real life public health settings including considerations of institutions, people, work practices, culture, politics, and other issues. The focus is on understanding informatics principles to population health with different levels of granularity going down to the level of the individual. In the rest of this chapter, we scope out our definition of PHI, its underlying principles, and emphasize what is included in this domain.

1.3.2 Computer science and informatics

We will now historically trace some developments in computer science, informatics, and then health informatics. While various developments which provide the foundations of computer science far predate the development of the digital computer, such as the building of Abacus and Pascal's calculator, the first computer only came into being in the 1940s. The academic field of computer science was established in the 1950s, when the University of Cambridge Computer Laboratory in the United Kingdom started the Cambridge Diploma in Computer Science in 1953. In North America, the first computer science degree programme was established about a decade later at Purdue University. Computer science represents the systematic study of algorithmic methods for representing and transforming information, including their theory, design, implementation, application, and efficiency. The roots of computer science extend deeply into mathematics and engineering; while the former imparts analysis, the latter provides for design inputs. Today, the academic field of computer science is well established, with significant achievements in a relatively short time which span about six decades.

Information systems, which first had its origins in computer science, has a different focus than its parent. It represents an academic study of systems with a specific reference to information and the complementary networks of hardware and software that people and organizations use to collect, filter, process, create, use, and also distribute data. It represents the information and communications technologies (ICTs) that an organization uses and the way in which people interact with this technology in support of different kinds of business processes. As an academic discipline, it emerged in the early 1970s in North America, where the first doctoral degree in the subject was awarded in a business school. The early influences on information systems naturally came from computer science, reflected in the initial emphasis on artificial intelligence, building expert systems for 'structured problems' such as playing chess and medical diagnosis, and attempts to replicate the brain. Limited success emerged from these efforts, which provided the impetus to the emerging of the field of information systems concerned with studying how computer-based applications could be made useful for business settings. Early applications were largely in domains of accounting and finance, since number crunching was an obvious application of computers. Many of the early information systems groups in universities were born in accounting departments, and some still continue to live on there, for example, in the Case Western University in Ohio, United States, the University of Alberta in Edmonton, Canada, and in the Business School in the University of Manchester, United Kingdom.

Towards the end of 1970s and early 1980s, a number of efforts were seen in North America to apply computer-based systems to various business domains such as sales, marketing, and human resources. The primary focus of these efforts was on building increasingly sophisticated technical systems. However, the realization slowly started to dawn that despite better technical systems, their impact on improved use of information and organizational systems remained limited. This led to a surge in interest in trying to understand the organizational factors (or their absence) that lead to the success or failure of systems. Among the factors identified included top management support, strategy, alignment of business and IT strategy, and the influences of conflict, culture, and politics. While the identification of these organizational and management factors were a step forward in the right direction over a primary focus on the technical systems, there were critiques to this approach. The concerns included that the approach tended to be static, ignoring the processual dynamics associated with information systems implementation; and was 'decontextualized', being limited in its ability to develop understanding of the linkages between context (the pre-existing conditions of the implementation settings), and the implementation dynamics of the system. This limited the generalizability of research findings, or the use of systems in multiple contexts, as each implementation context was unique and so the factors and processes would vary.

These critiques contributed to two broad shifts in information systems research. The first concerned a greater emphasis on the building of process-based understandings of how information systems are implemented in organizational settings. The second was to develop more social science-informed understandings of the relation between the 'social' and the 'technical', with Kling's 'web model' (Kling 1987) being a pioneering effort in this direction. Slowly, various social theories such as Giddens' structuration, and Foucault's power and control were introduced into information systems research to help understand issues of context, structure and agency, subjective meanings and inter-subjectivity, unintended consequences, and various others. As various social theories and associated methods came in to fashion, a rising concern was of the increased emphasis on the social aspects, and in the process ignoring and black-boxing the technology. This led to calls of 'taking technology seriously' and 'desperately seeking the technical artefact' (Orlikowski and Iacono 2001). From the early 2000s we also see an increasing emphasis on understanding the materiality of the technology and how this shapes human behaviour. Latour's Actor–Network Theory (ANT), which attributed symmetry of agency to technology and humans, and Information Infrastructure Theory, which builds upon ANT principles but applies them to the study of large-scale, complex, and inter-connected systems like the internet, were popular approaches that researchers drew upon.

Today, as the use of computers has become all-pervasive in almost all aspects of our everyday social and professional lives, the academic field of information systems struggles to position itself—as an entity of its own, or as a part of another discipline, or to be not explicit, as different departments build their own understanding and systems to support their particular domains of work. In North America, information systems is typically housed within Schools of Business, aligned more closely to the more IT proactive groups such as accounts, finance, or marketing. In the United Kingdom, where there seems to be gradual shrinking of the information systems field, the existing faculties have typically been merged with other departments, such as business (such as at Cambridge), management (such as at the London School of Economics), or accounting (e.g. Manchester). So, currently there exists a fair degree of ambiguity on where is the home of information systems, and, even more extreme— whether it should exist as a discipline or not. Echoing *Hamlet*, one may well exclaim ... 'To be or not to be—that is the question'.

How do these trends in research and academic information systems shape their development and use in practical settings? While these linkages are not obvious to trace, we can broadly infer that research tends to lag behind practice. For example, big data has for many years been an object of focus for consultants and for big corporations like Google and Amazon, but is only recently becoming a serious topic of research for most information systems academic groups in universities. From the health domain, the topics of civil registration and universal health coverage have been subject to serious discussion by global agencies like the World Health Organization (WHO) and World Bank for more than five years, and despite their significant information systems implications, have not yet been studied by informatics researchers. Further, research trends today start with building eulogies of new technologies, such as social media, mobile, and big data, followed by studies of attempts to apply them in organizational settings with often limited results, and then leading to increasingly sophisticated social science-based analysis of 'why' systems do not perform to their expected potential. More critically, it can be said that researchers have been developing more elegant ways of saying the same story of unrealized potential of ICTs in different settings, especially in the context of LMICs.

In summary, the fields of informatics and information systems have pursued different trajectories in North America and Europe, and have continued to grow significantly over the last four to five decades, but in different academic homes. A point to note is that in LMICs, despite being a dominant geography which hosts different types of ICT applications in business and government, the discipline of information systems does not find a place in the academic curriculum of most local educational institutions. The dominant focus in institutions here still continues to be computer science and IT, arguably keeping an eye on the employment potential of the global outsourcing market in countries like India and China, and the employment possibilities for the IT-skilled workforce in North America and the United Kingdom. Even in leading management and business schools in LMICs, the discipline of information systems is conspicuous by its absence. An important implication of this neglect is that while LMICs produce large numbers of IT-skilled persons, expertise in design and implementation informed by social science-based understandings is often much more limited. It is said of the Indian software industry, that while there are sharp skills available to design different pieces of a shirt, there is a lack of expertise to design and market the whole shirt. However, this situation is changing, with many of the Indian IT majors accumulating expertise to build products and take them to global markets. As a parallel, we see adequate skills available in health informatics, but not comparably in health information systems. This comment comes from collective observations the authors have developed over 20 years of research and practice, spanning more than 50 countries.

After this brief historical sketch of the field of computer science and informatics, we similarly trace the evolution of *health* informatics, with a focus towards LMICs.

1.3.3 A historical overview of developments in health informatics

Health informatics refers to both the practice of a speciality and a field of study, incorporating processes, theories, procedures, and concepts from computer and information sciences, health sciences (nursing and medical sciences), and also the social sciences (cognitive and organizational theory). Health informatics as a discipline can be traced back to the 1950s, initially characterized by experiments involving the application of computers to nursing and medicine, leading to the invention of the computed tomography (CT) scanner in the early seventies. The goals of health informatics are to support broadly the application of computers to improve healthcare delivery and health status. While computer science brings to health ·informatics the technology and software coding required for this speciality, information sciences contributes to the procedures and processes needed to develop and process data, information, and knowledge. Understanding the scope and boundaries of health informatics needs to begin with the appreciation of its roots in computers and information sciences.

The first computer came into being in the 1960s through IBM, and soon after, early efforts at automation began in the area of healthcare, and health informatics started to emerge as a new discipline. By the 1980s, the personal computer emerged and forever changed the nature of computing within the health domain. As healthcare providers increasingly became direct users of the computers, they began to discover various new uses for this technology, also contributing to tensions between centralized and decentralized models to support technology within healthcare settings.

Information science as a discipline investigates the properties and behaviour of information, the forces governing the flow of information, and the means of processing it for optimum usability and accessibility. Information science has evolved through the convergence and influence of various disciplines including library sciences, computer sciences, communication, and behavioural sciences. This includes the investigation of information representation in both natural and artificial systems, the use of codes for efficient message transmission, and the study of information processing devices and techniques, such as computers and other programming systems (Nelson and Staggers 2013).

1.3.4 Health informatics developments in high-income countries

In North America, health informatics is referred to by many names including healthcare informatics, medical informatics, nursing informatics, clinical informatics, or biomedical informatics. All broadly refer to a multidisciplinary field, including domains of computer science, information science, and behavioural sciences, concerned with applying informatics in healthcare, typically at the patient level. A key focus of these efforts has been towards strengthening efficiencies, reducing costs, identifying new opportunities, and improving clinical care for individuals. Establishing standards has been another key focus of this field, and in as far back as 1938, the American Association of Medical Record Librarians (AAMRL) and its members were known as medical record experts or librarians who studied medical record science. The goal was to raise the standards of record-keeping in hospitals and other healthcare facilities, and to guarantee accuracy and precision. Over time, the name of AAMRL changed to American Health Information Management Association (AHIMA) to reflect the wider variety of areas which health professionals work in today.

The tools focused on by American health informatics efforts include computers, clinical guidelines, formal medical terminologies, and other information and communication systems, applied to nursing, clinical care, dentistry, pharmacy, medical research, and others. A primary focus has been on the development of electronic health records (EHRs) to be used in hospitals. Primary healthcare systems that are population based have been largely ignored in this path of development. Homer Warner is credited with being one of the fathers of medical informatics, and for founding the Department of Medical Informatics at the University of Utah in 1968. Today many universities host academic programmes in the area, such as Idaho State, Kent State, Drexel, and the University of Illinois. Furthermore, various other informatics certifications are provided, in nursing, radiology, and imaging for example. Since the 1960s and 1970s, the speciality has grown rapidly with the publication of various books, the development of new journals, the establishment of various professional organizations, and creation of university-led educational and certification programmes.

Historically, the EHR has been continually expressed as an evolution of health record-keeping and a subject of extensive debate with regard to factors related to access and privacy among the health professional community. This focus is also currently evident in great force, beginning with President George Bush's efforts to establish the National Health Information Network (NHIN), efforts which were subsequently reinforced by President Obama who emphasized the importance of big data technologies, and initiated efforts such as *My Data, Open Data, and Data.gov* where people can access public data that is secured and available in real time. The government emphasized changes in existing laws to accommodate the new needs of security and privacy, supported by the Health Insurance Portability and Accountability Act (HIPAA) of 1996 and the Safe Harbour Act. These actions have been authorized by the Health Information Technology for Economic and Clinical Health (HITECH) Act, part of the American Recovery and Reinvestment Act of 2009, also known as the Stimulus Bill. The HITECH Act included four sets of interventions: defining of meaningful use; encouragement and support for attainment of meaningful use through incentives and grant programmes; bolstering public trust in EHRs by ensuring their privacy and security; and fostering continued health IT innovation. In practice, the implementation challenges of these initiatives have extended beyond information and technical support and included issues of acquisition and maintenance costs, lack of capital for small healthcare providers, and concerns about loss of productivity and income during the implementation and learning phases. Arguably, and in summary, the EHR which was the initial focus of health informatics efforts in North America continues to be so, with more vigour, in a much bigger form (of a national architecture), and supported by an extensive policy, regulatory, and financial infrastructure.

Canada too has embarked on a large-scale health IT blueprint called Infoway, representing a form of 'open health architecture'. At the heart of this blueprint is the development of a large centralized EHR, which has also been taken up by countries like the United Kingdom, and also some LMICs like Rwanda under their 'Rwanda Health Information Exchange' initiative. These efforts have met with serious criticisms (National Audit Office 2011). Webster (2011) has argued that Canada should revisit its EHR strategy as it is wasteful and flawed. These critiques are also reflected by reports from the United Kingdom on their efforts, which have been described as not practical or achievable. Norm Archer, Professor Emeritus at McMaster University in Hamilton, Ontario, has written 'They should not try to implement it (EHRs) in the short term. To set out with a highly centralized system and try to extend it downwards [towards patients and clinicians] doesn't work' (Webster 2011). Archer worries that Infoway (used in Canada) may have locked itself into its vision and current approach towards the development of EHRs as a result of signing contracts with IT firms. A large percentage of the Infoway investments have been in large IT systems, and only 17 per cent of its $2.1 billion in outlays since 2001 is earmarked for clinician-level implementation. Archer notes that the bigger the project, the less likely it is to be successful, and Infoway has delivered disappointing results—and blueprints for an EHR available nationwide 'anywhere, anytime in support of high quality care', is highly likely to fail. The Auditor General of Canada has criticized Canadian information technology procurement, most recently in the Status Report of the Auditor General of Canada (2011).

In the United Kingdom, the growth of health informatics has followed a slightly different trajectory than in North America, but has had EHR at the centre of its efforts, as typified by the following statement:

> 'We will put patients at the heart of the NHS, through an information revolution and greater choice and control with shared decision-making becoming the norm: "no decision about me without me" and patients having access to the information they want, to make choices about their care. They will have increased control over their own care records'

(Department of Health UK 2010, p. 3.)

The UK health informatics community has long played a key role in international activity, joining TC4 of the International Federation of Information Processing (1969), which later became IMIA (1979). Hayes and Barnett (2008) described the path taken by the United Kingdom with respect to the development of health informatics as initially unorganized and idiosyncratic, dominated by concerns of finance, and subsequently including solutions for pathology, radiotherapy, immunization, and primary care. Many of these solutions, even in the early 1970s, were developed in-house by experts in the field to meet their particular requirements and were largely individual-focused. The coalition government in 2010 proposed a return to the strategy of equity and excellence, providing a significant opportunity for health informaticians to come out of the back office and take up a frontline role in supporting clinical practice.

There have been various criticisms made to the UK efforts for developing a central EHR. A UK Public Administration Select Committee report, *Government and IT—'a recipe for rip-offs': time for a new approach*, concluded that the government essentially does not know how to develop IT systems or judiciously shop for either hardware or software. 'IT procurement has too often resulted in late, over budget IT systems that are not fit for purpose', states the report (Webster 2011). The UK Department of Health has already spent roughly £2.7 billion on its electronic medical records plan, with the bulk of the money having been awarded to major software firms such as Accenture, Fujitsu, Computer Sciences Corporation, and BT Software. This has created a small oligopoly of large suppliers, representing a 'cartel' leading to a perverse situation in which governments have wasted significant amounts of public money, and of procurement at substantially higher rates than the commercial market. These criticisms are similar to those made against the Canada Health Infoway, and that large-scale national EHRs are likely to be less efficient, cost-effective, or safe, and contain less trusted information than smaller, more local systems. Such 'eye-catching' large systems tend to be the product of a top-down enthusiast-driven approach, which are crafted with 'insufficient engagement of clinical users'. Dipak Kalra, Professor of Health Informatics at University College, London, has described the UK approach as 'over-ambitious in areas where there was little evidence and no experience to build upon' (Webster 2011). There is limited transparency to the procurements, as the Crown corporation is not subject to financial disclosure rules that obligate it to disclose contracts or salary information.

Neither the UK's Department of Health nor Prime Minister David Cameron's government has responded to the Parliamentary calls for the jettisoning of Britain's EHR initiative. But the Department of Health said in response to a scathing National Audit Office report, *The National Programme for IT in the NHS: an update on the delivery of detailed care records systems* that its investments 'will potentially deliver value for money' because reforms to the 'future architecture of the programme' will allow 'many sources of information to be connected together as opposed to assuming that all relevant information will be stored in a single system'.

France has learned the lesson of the follies of large, centralized EHRs, and has recently abandoned its plans, notes Karl Stroetmann, author of a recent pan-European survey of e-health progress commissioned by the European Commission (Stroetmann *et al.* 2011). 'They made little progress and have now stopped the whole project', he says, 'They're starting again from scratch'.

Summarizing the experiences from the high-income countries, it can be seen that centralized, large-scale EHRs have been the focus of national level health informatics efforts, but to date have yielded minimum results. These experiences have highlighted the value of going for low-cost, locally driven efforts. A population-based and use focus is noticeably absent in these EHR efforts, as the individual patient is given primary attention, without the functionality to be able to roll it up to the level of populations and public health.

1.4 Health Informatics Developments in Low and Middle-Income Countries

This domain of health informatics has been largely absent in most LMICs with a few exceptions, such as in China and Brazil. In China, a key focus has been on hospital information systems, aimed at minimizing unnecessary waste and repetition, and subsequently promoting the efficiency and quality-control of healthcare. By 2004, China had successfully spread their hospital information systems through approximately 35–40 per cent of nationwide hospitals, with a high degree of regional variations, with the east being far ahead than the north. China has been greatly improving its health informatics since it finally joined the World Trade Organization (WTO), and is simultaneously also improving its higher education. At the end of 2002, there were 77 medical universities and medical colleges in China, and 48 of these offered Bachelor's, Master's, and Doctorate degrees in medicine. In 2003, Severe Acute Respiratory Syndrome (SARS) played a large role in the rapid improving of the healthcare system, with the hospital information system being swiftly expanded to cover 80 per cent of hospitals. Comparisons with the Korean healthcare system have also spurred the Chinese to strengthen their health informatics component.

Similarly, in Brazil, the first applications of computers to medicine and healthcare started in around 1968, with the installation of the first mainframes in public university hospitals for supporting the hospital census in the School of Medicine of Ribeirao Preto and patient master files in the Hospital das Clinicas da Universidade de Sao Paulo. In the 1970s, several hospitals acquired computers for various units such as intensive care, cardiology, diagnostics, and patient monitoring. In the early 1980s, with the arrival of cheaper personal computers

(PCs), a great upsurge of computer applications in health ensued, and in 1986 the Brazilian Society of Health Informatics was founded, the first Brazilian Congress of Health Informatics was held, and the first *Brazilian Journal of Health Informatics* was published. In Brazil, two universities (University of Sao Paulo and Federal University of Sao Paulo) offer undergraduate and post-graduate programmes in medical informatics.

There are limited other examples noted in LMICs regarding the institutional development of health informatics as a field of academic specialization in established educational institutions. This is despite the fact that in nations like India, Thailand, or South Africa, the introduction and use of health informatics products in their top private corporate hospitals was usually on par with that in the hospitals of developed nations. This is similar to the difference between importing the latest car or MRI machine, and being able to design and deploy one. However, there have been significant developments taking place in informatics for primary healthcare in LMICs.

While as an academic discipline the field of health informatics has not really evolved in LMICs, tremendous experience has been generated in the practice of building systems to support primary healthcare, largely population-based efforts through national routine systems, for specific programmes such as immunization, mother and child health, tuberculosis (TB), and Human Immunodeficiency Virus (HIV). Since the 1980s, various LMICs have made reform of these information systems as an integral component of their health system strengthening efforts, supported by strong donor investments. However, the potential of these IT projects has been largely untapped, and Heeks (2002) has noted that about 90 per cent of such efforts have been complete or partial failures. However, this has not deterred governments and donors. On the contrary, efforts have accelerated, especially in the last 5 to 10 years.

Various global initiatives have contributed to this increased interest in IT for health projects. One significant effort was by the Health Metrics Network (HMN), set up in 2006 as a Secretariat of the WHO to help countries develop and implement national strategies for the strengthening of systems. HMN developed a framework based on principles of data warehousing, which sought to create common repositories of shared data that could satisfy the information needs of a wide range of stakeholders, rather than developing individual stand-alone systems for particular programmes or departments. This data warehousing approach, drawn from the enterprise architecture framework and geared to addressing the problem of fragmentation of information systems, achieved significant success in the short lifespan of HMN. Many countries developed strategies and started implementation of such models. Some countries like Sierra Leone made significant advances, also becoming a role model for other countries in West Africa. However, much longer-term efforts and support were needed to enable full fruition of the HMN initiative, which did not happen.

Traditionally health informatics deals with a diverse range of systems including health management information systems (HMIS), EHRs, clinical decision support systems (CDSS), laboratory information systems (LIS), radiology information systems (RIS), picture archiving and communication systems (PACS), Telehealth, and various others. LMICs largely have subsystems of public health information systems for health administration support, district health management, hospital management, procurement, and logistics support (for drugs and other supplies), human resources management systems, geographic information systems for health, disease surveillance, emergency response support, healthcare financing systems, and various others. These different systems have varying supporting infrastructure and platforms. Such systems could be of little or no interest to clinicians per se—but public health management increasingly depends on such systems and cannot do without it.

New technologies are often positioned as silver bullets to solve problems that are necessarily health or institutionally related. The extensive deployment of mHealth (mobile health) applications and the resulting 'pilotitis' reflects efforts which die as small-scale pilots. While web-based deployment of systems is increasingly becoming the norm in many LMICs, there are institutional considerations of ownership, access, and data regulation which are matters of intense debate, some of which we take up in this book. From the perspective of institutional and technological conditions in LMICs, considered design choices are required which can account for the diversity of media and platforms, and where paper often remains the dominant one. Another key aspect of the informatics positioning concerns the discussions on standards. While medical standards like SNOMED CT and HL7 are becoming widespread, their relevance cannot be ignored by LMICs, as they carry various political and commercial dimensions. Public health systems are also engaging with more routine standards concerning nomenclature, formats, and periodicities. Building understanding of these different standards, and how they relate (or not) to each other will be an important focus of reform efforts in the future.

Today, the scenario with respect to health IT has changed dramatically with the proliferation of new tools such as web technologies, mobile devices, other forms of data entry devices, cloud computing, and improved models for technical integration. The growth of open source software solutions helps countries to avoid lock-ins to large-scale and failed proprietary-based systems, and experiment with relatively lesser risks. Web-based systems, based on open source software, have been instrumental in enabling countries like Ghana and Kenya to develop national scale HMIS. These developments have been made possible through access to cloud computing, an issue which we discuss in detail in Chapter 5.

Now many LMICs are experimenting with different forms of name-based or individually focused systems. India has developed a mother and child tracking system (MCTS) for tracking pregnant mothers from the time of their first ante-natal registration, through different stages of their care including delivery and postnatal care. This MCTS is also designed for child immunization, to track by name of the child the vaccination cycle from the first dose to full immuniza-tion. In Ghana, there is a line listing application being used to register births, although only to record the events, not to track them. In Tajikistan, there are ongoing efforts to create a system to register all civil registration events of births and deaths. Many countries are seeking to track individual TB or HIV cases. This shift to the use and tracking of systems based on names raises vari-ous new and unexplored issues, including those related to system design, inte-gration, governance, data privacy, security, and infrastructure requirements. Furthermore, while there is an explosion of data which becomes available, the capacity to use it is not growing in the same manner. In subsequent chapters, we will try to explore these issues from a PHI perspective in order to under-stand how to shape research and practice.

In summary, most LMICs have made significant progress in the last decade on strengthening their systems in support of primary care systems, which are primarily aggregate and population based. Efforts to strengthen individual-based systems at the community level through recording and tracking are typi-cally at a nascent stage, with limited ability to be aggregated to a population base. The focus on EHRs has been largely absent in most LMICs, but is likely to grow in the future. While efforts in practice are rapidly evolving, academic studies in health informatics in LMICs is not moving at a comparable pace.

1.5 Summarizing Trends in Informatics and Health Informatics

In summary, in high-income countries, the primary orientation of health infor-matics is towards medical informatics, with the focus being on the individual and the supporting EHR. Primary healthcare systems with a focus on popula-tions tend to be de-emphasized in relation to curative individual patient-based care. Many of the systems have been developed by medical practitioners for themselves. This focus contributes to building a strongly positivistic academic orientation, drawn from the origin of the field in the domains of computers, information, and medical sciences, which marginalizes the understanding of the population and context. In LMICs, while the focus has been primarily on the practice of strengthening systems for primary healthcare, the academic discipline to support these efforts has lagged far behind. Studies have been focused on medicine or technology, without trying to understand the inter-linkages in context. Some overall trends are briefly discussed.

1.5.1 Primary orientation towards health and medical informatics

In North America, United Kingdom, and other rich countries, the origin of health informatics is intimately tied up with the growth in computer technol-ogy, information, and behavioural sciences. The arrival of the computer, and the PC in particular, contributed to a surge in health informatics applications in different aspects of healthcare, notably nursing, clinical care, radiology, and others. The EHR or the individual patient record has been a key focus of sta-tus to measure progress in health informatics efforts. The current US govern-ment's efforts (2016) to establish a national architecture for EHR, supported under the HITECH Act, reflects this evolution both in terms of creating a more sophisticated inter-connected architecture of national scale, and a supporting legal and regulatory environment. Even in the United Kingdom, the primary focus of the medical informatics efforts has been largely geared towards hos-pital information systems and the associated EHR. Another characteristic of these efforts has been that the systems have been largely developed by in-house experts such as clinicians and other health technicians. This is probably indica-tive of the lack of collaborative efforts between the health and informatics com-munities, contributing to a bias towards small-scale systems being developed for individual use, which constrain systems thinking and design of broader 'health information architectures' (Sahay and Braa 2012). The focus towards building large-scale EHR systems, such as in Canada and the United Kingdom, has yielded not so positive results. This individual-based focus has contributed to increased fragmentation of systems and an absence of a population-based approach. For example, the Norwegian University Research Hospital is cur-rently trying to harmonize a fragmented silo portfolio of more than 800 dif-ferent systems, and over 2500 in the south east region (Bygstad and Hanseth 2015), which have been built over time to suit particular information needs of doctors and their respective specializations.

1.5.2 Strongly positivistic orientation towards practice and academics of health informatics

Given that the primary impetus for both the practice and study of health informatics came from computer science, information science, and cognitive psychology, the orientation of practice and academia has been largely based on principles of positivism. Such a focus tends to study the relation between independent and dependent variables, creating correlations, and their statistical generalizations to larger populations. Doctors and technicians, with primary educational training in medicine and its allied fields like imaging and radiology, by design are embedded in such a positivistic focus. This has implied a primary focus on measurement and improving efficiencies relating to clinical care and drug trials. Even the principles of Taylor's scientific management were explicitly applied to improve healthcare in North America, based on principles of positivism (Rastegar 2004).

1.5.3 Neglect of informatics for primary healthcare systems in rich countries

With the primary focus of health informatics being on the individual patient through hospital information systems and EHR, systems for primary healthcare with a primary focus on populations have naturally been neglected. As an academic discipline as well, primary healthcare and its supporting information systems have been largely neglected. In richer countries like Norway, where primary healthcare is organized through the systems of general practitioners with limited obligations for national reporting, population-based systems have not found significant focus. The systems of disease registries established in Norway, for example, are used more to guide research efforts than for strengthening public health systems.

1.5.4 Neglect of low and middle-income countries in the study of health informatics evolution

The history of health informatics as an academic discipline is a product of the Western world, in which LMICs find little to no mention. The exceptions in this regard are China and Brazil, which have also focused primarily on hospital-based information systems with a focus on EHRs. However, and in contrast, the practice of applying IT to primary healthcare systems has evolved significantly in LMICs over the last two decades. Now as countries are reaching higher levels of data collection coverage and quality, there is an increasing focus being placed on how this data can be used to improve the health of populations. There are initial forays being made into the development of name-based systems for programme tracking and events recording, but they are still in a nascent stage, especially in their ability to be aggregated to population-based systems, and integration with other routine reporting systems. There has been a conscious neglect of hospital information systems and EHRs in these public information systems, but they are expected to receive increased focus in the future.

Given these trends in the evolution of health informatics, we conclude in the final section with a case for a more 'expanded public health informatics' (we refer to this later as 'Expanded PHI') focus in LMICs.

1.6 A Case For a More Expanded Public Health Informatics Focus in Low and Middle-Income Countries

The discussions in section 1.5, *Summarizing Trends in Informatics and Health Informatics*, have broadly emphasized a patient-centric approach to health informatics being dominant in rich counties, and a more population-based primary health approach being evident in LMICs. These two streams have largely excluded the other, both in practice and academia. Our book is about trying to develop an 'expanded public health informatics' approach that transcends both these kinds of systems, with the unifying element being an interest in strengthening population-based health systems. So, this will involve design approaches which allow individual systems to be aggregated to a population-based one, and the ability to drill down from aggregate systems to individuals to help prioritize action where it is needed most. However, to this end, two disconnects are currently evident: one, between developments in the West and those in LMICs; and two, between practice and academics within LMICs.

While health informatics has grown by leaps and bounds since the 1960s, and with increasing pace in the last couple of decades, such growth has been limited in LMICs. Academia in LMICs lags significantly behind practice, with few exceptions. Brazil and China have shown growth in both practice and academics, but with a primary focus on hospital-based information systems and EHRs, as is also the case in the rich countries. Various LMICs have embarked on strengthening their HMIS, including the collection and processing of routine aggregate data, and transmitting them from the periphery through various administrative levels of the district, province, and national levels. Various books, papers, and PhD theses have been written by scholars (mostly based in Western universities) on the subject, with limited outputs coming from local in-country scholars. Academic institutions in LMICs have so far not engaged in the study of such systems in their contexts, resulting in practice far outpacing academia.

In studying national HMIS implementation efforts through their HISP (Health Information Systems Programme) research and development initiative, the efforts of the Department of Informatics, University of Oslo, Norway, are significant. HISP as a research programme was born in 1994 in South Africa, supported by Norwegian State funds. HISP was bathed in the Scandinavian action research tradition and had four inter-connected components: one, research into the design, development, and implementation of HMIS in LMICs; two, the design, development and support of open source HMIS software called DHIS (District Health Information Software—http://www.dhis2.org) at national and lower levels in countries; three, establish a Master's programme in health informatics; and finally, PhD research involving LMIC scholars registering for academic work in Oslo, and studying problems germane to their respective countries. Through these respective inter-connected efforts, now spanning more than two decades, Oslo has established collaborative Master's programmes with universities in Mozambique, Malawi, Tanzania, South Africa, Ethiopia, and Sri Lanka. There is a full Master's programme in health information systems being offered by the University of Gadjah Mada, Yogyakarta in Indonesia. Other than these, there are no fully established Master's courses in this subject specifically in and for LMICs. However, various universities in LMICs are trying to establish single courses or modules within public health Master's programmes and sometimes within informatics.

Our direct experience in engaging with the Oslo-collaborated educational programmes has helped us to understand the tremendous demand for health informatics in LMICs, which spans at least the disciplines of public health and informatics, and the need for a 'health information systems' framing. The high number of efforts with computerization ongoing in most LMICs creates an urgent need to strengthen the national educational base, which can contribute to strengthening the national autonomy and ownership of systems, and simultaneously reduce crippling levels of donor dependence. From an academic perspective, health informatics provides for a unique subject of study currently ignored by universities.

1.7 **Conclusions**

In this chapter, we have developed the argument for the need to articulate an Expanded PHI perspective to guide health informatics strengthening efforts— both research and practice—in LMICs.

While health informatics is an area of specialization for applications of computer-based technology in healthcare, the question of which discipline it falls into has never been definitively established. It has been variably perceived as a speciality within computer science, or within information science, or within various healthcare disciplines notably public health, or as an interdisciplinary healthcare facility. We argue that this Expanded PHI perspective need not be rooted in specific historical roots of its parent disciplines and practices, but be developed by creating a hybrid across levels of research, practice, and focus. This does not make the PHI perspective only about either healthcare or informatics, but they are to be combined and more, to create a new form of hybridized knowledge, which has population health as a unifying focus.

After raising the need for the development of a PHI focus in the context of LMICs, in Chapter 2 we position this within a public health framework. Combining arguments from both informatics and public health, we then, in subsequent chapters, develop design principles to analyse problematic issues of integration, use of information, governance, and others which represent contemporary challenges for this domain.

1.8 **References**

Auditor General of Canada (2011). Status Report. [Online]. Available at: http://www.oag-bvg.gc.ca/internet/English/parl_oag_201106_02_e_35370.html [Last accessed: 1 October 2015].

Bygstad, B. and **Hanseth, O.** (2015). From IT Silos to Integrated Solutions: A Study in E-health Complexity. *ECIS 2015 Completed Research Papers*, Paper 23.

Department of Health UK (2010). *Equity and Excellence: Liberating the NHS*. Stationary Office, London, UK.

Hayes, G. and **Barnett, D.** (2008). *UK Health Computing: Recollections and Reflections*. British Computer Society, Swindon, UK.

Heeks, R. (2002). Information systems and developing countries: Failure, success, and local improvisations. *The Information Society*, 18(2), 101–12.

Kling, R. (1987). Defining the boundaries of computing across complex organizations. In: **Hirschheim, R.A** (ed.). *Critical Issues in Information Systems Research*. John Wiley & Sons, Inc., New York, NY.

National Audit Office, UK (2011). The National Programme for IT in the NHS: an update on the delivery of detailed care records systems [Online]. Available at: http://www.nao.org.uk/report/the-national-programme-for-it-in-the-nhs-an-update-on-the-delivery-of-detailed-care-records-systems [Last accessed: 1 October 2015].

Nelson, R. and **Staggers, N.** (2013). *Health Informatics: An Interprofessional Approach*. Elsevier Health Sciences, St Louis, MO.

Orlikowski, W.J. and **Iacono, C.S.** (2001). Research commentary: Desperately seeking the 'IT' in IT research—A call to theorizing the IT artifact. *Information systems research*, 12(2), 121–34.

Rastegar, D.A. (2004). Health care becomes an industry. *The Annals of Family Medicine*, 2(1), 79–83.

Sahay S. and **Braa, J.** (2012). *Integrated Health Information Architecture. Power to the Users: Design, Development and Use*. Matrix Publishers, New Delhi, India, pp. 148–9.

Stroetmann K., Artmann, J., Stroetmann V.N., *et al.* (2011). European countries on their journey towards national eHealth infrastructures. *European Commission Information Society*. [Online]. Available at: http://www.ehealthnews.eu/images/stories/pdf/ehstrategies_final_report.pdf [Last accessed: 1 October 2015].

Webster, P.C. (2011). Centralized, nationwide electronic health records schemes under assault. *Canadian Medical Association Journal*, 183(15), 1105–6.

Chapter 2

Understanding Public Health Informatics in Context of Health in Low and Middle-Income Countries

2.1 Public Health Informatics in the Context of Health in Low and Middle-Income Countries

This chapter builds upon the first one. Chapter 1 situated public health informatics (PHI) in a historical perspective to understand how computers, and technical and medical biases have shaped the trajectory of PHI, leading to the neglect of focus on public health issues, especially in the context of LMICs.

This chapter attempts to situate PHI in the context of public health in LMICs, which will lead to the articulation of an integrated PHI perspective that combines understandings from the informatics and public health domains.

2.2 Defining Public Health

'Public Health is the science and the art of preventing disease, prolonging life, and promoting physical health and efficiency through organised community efforts for the sanitation of the environment, the control of community infections, the education of the individual in principles of personal hygiene, the organisation of medical and nursing services for the early diagnosis and preventive treatment of disease, and the development of the social machinery which will ensure to every individual in the community a standard of living adequate for the maintenance of health'

(Winslow 1920).

The distinction of public health from medical care is important to grasp. Medical care is often used interchangeably with healthcare, and relates largely to the prevention, diagnosis, and management of disease in an individual patient, typically within a clinical establishment like a hospital. In contrast, public health is concerned with *the health of populations*. The mission statement of John Hopkins Bloomberg School of Public Health expresses this quite lucidly as 'Protecting Health, Saving Lives—Millions at a Time' (http://www.jhsph.edu/about/).

Sometimes public health refers only to preventive and promotive aspects of health, and excludes clinical care. Preventive and promotive care can take the form of action of other non-health sectors, like the impact of air pollution on health, the provision of safe drinking water, or of preventive health services like immunization or vector control. While promotive and preventive care are undoubtedly important components, the scope of public health is not limited to these. Public health also includes the organization of curative or clinical healthcare services to ensure access, equity, affordability, and quality of medical care services.

Another important statement of the goals of public health is the historic Declaration of Alma-Ata of 1978. This declaration, one of the most important public health documents of all times, defines health 'as a state of complete physical, mental and social well-being, and not merely the absence of disease or infirmity'. It further elaborates that health is a fundamental right and that the attainment of this is a most important world-wide social goal. Alma-Ata established primary healthcare as the key strategy to the achievement of health for all.

An important unifying theme in all these definitions is that the object is not the single individual or family, but a population; and information on healthcare of many individuals is translated to issues of health status, equity, access, and the quality of care enjoyed by all. This has important implications for PHI, as we will go on to argue in this chapter. First, we discuss the primary healthcare component in more detail.

2.3 **Public Health and Primary Healthcare**

A term closely related to public health, which again implies multiple meanings, is that of 'primary healthcare'. One of the most accepted definitions of it is from the Alma-Ata Declaration: 'Primary healthcare is essential healthcare based on practical, scientifically sound and socially acceptable methods and technology made universally accessible to individuals and families in the community through their full participation and at a cost that the community and country can afford ... It is the first level of contact of individuals, the family and the community with the national health system, bringing healthcare as close as possible to where people live and work ...' (WHO 1978, Declaration VI).

The difference and overlap between public health and primary healthcare is important. In the context of LMICs, most countries are aspiring only for the realization of the more limited goal of comprehensive primary healthcare— thus de-emphasizing the focus on tertiary hospital care and consultations. Secondary care, including hospitalization, is however very much part of the usage. Thus, in its World Health Report of 2008, the WHO (World Health

Organization) points out that in low resource settings, primary care teams must be seen as a coordinating hub of a system where the district hospital is at the apex of a pyramid of primary care facilities (WHO 2008, p. 55). However, this de-emphasis on tertiary systems seems to be changing given the increasing global focus on universal health coverage and the emphasis of the latter on insurance systems for increasing both access to care and financial protection. Insurance-based financing is generally centred far more, or even exclusively, on hospital care as distinct from primary care. In either approach it becomes important to aggregate information of individuals seeking care at multiple sites into measures of population-based coverage, and vice versa—to move from only reporting aggregate numbers to providing more space for individual patient records.

There are many reasons why primary care is accorded this level of importance in most LMICs. Even in many high-income nations, there is a designated primary care provider for every individual and family. The reasons for such focus on primary healthcare as the key national health strategy include:

i)   A primary healthcare team understands the needs of its defined community and so is able to provide comprehensive, integrated, and patient-centred care.

ii) Comprehensive primary healthcare potentially provides value for money, that is, higher health outcomes at lower per capita total health expenditure. Such care would significantly reduce morbidity and mortality of the population at much lower costs to the system and the individual than a purely hospital-centric curative approach.

iii) The primary healthcare system serves an important referral function. Referral is both upwards to the specialists in secondary and tertiary based services, with primary healthcare acting as the channel of access to the latter, and then back from the specialist to the primary healthcare system, to provide follow-up care and access to affordable medication. Building these two-way referral linkages has implications on the informatics solutions, in terms of the content of information, its periodicity, and the amount of detail that needs to be circulated across levels.

2.4 **A Health Systems Understanding of Public Health**

This section addresses the question of what it takes to organize healthcare services within a more holistic understanding of the interlinkages discussed in section 2.3. The present way to answer this question is to see healthcare as a 'health system' made up of many inter-connected parts. The schematic diagram (see Fig. 2.1) articulated by the WHO visualizes this in the following manner.

THE WHO HEALTH SYSTEM FRAMEWORK

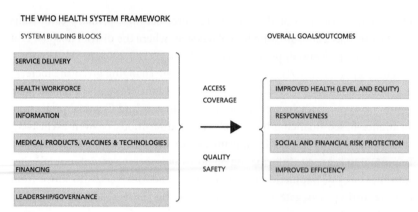

Fig. 2.1 The World Health Organization's framework for action.

Reproduced with permission from WHO, *Everybody's Business: Strengthening health systems to improve health outcomes—WHO's framework for action*. Geneva, World Health Organization, Copyright © 2007 WHO. Available from http://www.who.int/healthsystems/strategy/everybodys_business.pdf, accessed 01 Feb. 2016.

Though each of these components have been described as pillars, it would be more appropriate to picture them as a mesh by including inter-connections between these components. In other words, the system is much more than the sum of its parts, and represents a direction defined by its overall goals. The system has important values as attributes, including equity in access, quality of care, safety, patient autonomy and privacy, financial protection, and reaching the poorest and the most marginalized.

The outcomes are related to populations, and the system is thus constituted by the entire chain of hospitals, primary care facilities, and other healthcare activities which together provide healthcare services to populations. In many nations a significant part of this network of service providers is under public ownership, with varying levels of private care involvement. The measures of performance of a public healthcare system thus differ considerably from that of a single hospital or healthcare facility, which are individually focused on clinical care. However, the former (hospital derived information) is included in the latter (population-based information)! We argue that the public health perspective we are advocating should need to cover both primary and secondary and tertiary care services, and also their interlinkages.

The users of PHI would therefore differ from a perspective that is focused only on domains under clinical health informatics, or on aggregate reporting of selective primary healthcare data. The main users of PHI would be the public health manager of an administrative unit, along with facility managers of both hospitals and primary healthcare facilities, and also service providers at community levels. Policy makers would also need this information, as would community representatives, though with different information needs. In contrast, a sole focus on health informatics is understood as equivalent to biomedical informatics, clinical and medical imaging, with the users being the service providers and the individual patient, and secondarily the hospital management and insurance companies. The PHI perspective includes these users, but shifts the focus and emphasis to be able to link it to populations.

2.5 Information Needs of Public Health Systems: Transcending Primary and Medical Care Domains

While the information needs of a public health system were being fulfilled even before the era of information and communications technologies (ICTs), their introduction through the 1980s and 1990s and their rapid evolution in terms of databases, servers, mobile devices, open source systems, and various others, has been a major game changer in redefining information needs, the level and mechanisms by which these are met (or not), and the generation of new needs. While in the 1980s most LMIC health systems administrators were satisfied with aggregate data on reproductive and child health services, reported on a quarterly basis from the districts, today the demand is for patient level, longitudinal data on every transaction including the cost of patient care, within the perception of health system performance as understood by the universal health coverage discourse. This data is collected through a multiplicity of devices including mobiles, tablets, computers, scanners, and various others, and made available through many sources, including servers located in distant lands. There are thus some information needs that, being fulfilled earlier through paper forms, can now be done much faster, much easier, and with greater reliability. Furthermore, there are some information needs that were not attempted or addressed earlier, because it was not practical to gather this data or make necessary conclusions, but now ICTs makes it feasible. Thus, there are new possibilities for action that ICT-enhanced availability of information and its frequency have created.

In addition, there are multiple sources of information, which are being tapped for integration into different levels of management. These include routine reporting systems from the primary healthcare sector, electronic medical record systems in hospitals, surveys, surveillance sites, census, civil registration systems, and various others. PHI managers thus need to first understand the different information needs for public health, the available sources of information, and to which stakeholders should what information be made available, and in what form. Current discussions on big data, which includes data from various new kinds of sources, such as social media, genomics, Internet of Things, handheld devices and various others, provide new dimensions to information needs and sources. Health systems are still, however, grappling with the question of how some of these can be leveraged.

The data sources framework of the Health Metrics Network (HMN 2008) provides us a useful guideline to understand different facets of information needs (see Fig. 2.2). In this we include contemporary developments in big data while acknowledging that they currently represent untapped potential for public health.

However, we caution that the HMN data source framework shown can be misleading, because some of the priority services health service records are also population based. This is especially true of primary healthcare services, such as antenatal care and immunization, which are almost always population based. Pregnant women, infants, and other target populations are identified in a given service area, targets for coverage are set, and outreach services seek to reach the entire population. For example, registers of pregnant women and infants, as they are being maintained by field level nurses in the subcentres in India, are, in our view, examples of data sources and information systems that are better understood as being population based. While in a traditional health informatics perspective they may all be regarded as records from health services, in the PHI perspective, it is useful to emphasize that primary healthcare

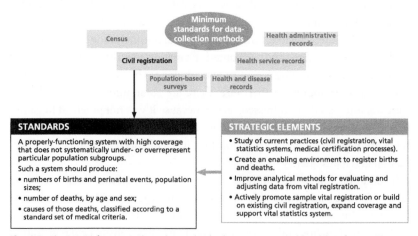

Fig. 2.2 The HMN framework and standards data sources and health information systems.

Reproduced with permission from Health Metrics Network, *Health Metrics Network: Framework and Standards for the Development of Country Health Information Systems*, Second Edition. Geneva, World Health Organization, Copyright © 2008 WHO. Available from http://apps.who.int/iris/bitstream/10665/43872/1/9789241595940_eng.pdf, accessed 01 Feb. 2016.

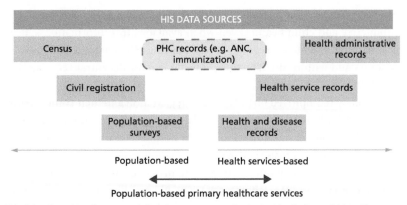

Fig. 2.3 The HMN framework for data sources adapted to include and identify records and registers from population-based primary healthcare services as population-based data sources.

Adapted with permission from Health Metrics Network, *Health Metrics Network: Framework and Standards for the Development of Country Health Information Systems*, Second Edition. Geneva, World Health Organization, Copyright © 2006 WHO. Available from http://apps.who.int/iris/bitstream/10665/43872/1/9789241595940_eng.pdf, accessed 01 Feb. 2016.

services could be considered as population-based health services in terms of information system development and data quality issues, as will be discussed later in this chapter. In Figure 2.3 we have amended the HMN data source framework to distinguish and include PHC records as population-based and as health services-based data sources. Though currently available only for ante-natal care (ANC) and immunization with universal health coverage, this same approach could extend to non-communicable diseases like hypertension and diabetes too (Fig. 2.3).

Using this framework, we discuss some domains of information needs within the context of public health, including different sources, spanning both primary care and medical care.

2.6 Understanding Health Status: Sourcing Real Time Morbidity and Mortality Data

For organizing services delivery, be it preventive or curative care, the first and foremost need is to have a good understanding of morbidity and mortality patterns; and epidemiological information concerning the prevalence on disease and its determinants. Public systems, especially in LMICs are resource constrained, raising the need to prioritize and plan, for which such information is essential. Until recently, epidemiological information in most LMICs was available from occasional and costly surveys, like the Demographic and

Health Surveys which typically covered very few indicators mostly related to reproductive and child health. Even when available, this information is usually at national and at best regional levels, but when there is such major diversity across and within districts, this is insufficient for decentralized planning and action.

However, with improved birth and death registration and their computerization, the establishment of disease surveillance programmes with the ability to draw up data from private and public sector hospitals on inpatient admissions and consultation diagnosis, and with information from registers of primary care providers (including information about drugs consumption patterns and diagnostic test results from laboratories), it would now become possible to provide much better morbidity and mortality information on a real time basis. We now have the power to triangulate data from multiple sources, improving the reliability and quality of data. Such information is usually in the form of rates and proportions, and the electronic health record or patient names and identification are seldom required.

The key challenge is that without integrating information from the many levels and sites of service provision and triangulating it with a good cause-of-death data of the civil registrations system, we would not have adequate information on morbidity, mortality, and the burden of disease. Data from primary healthcare programmes, for example, would give us population-based incidence and prevalence rates for most chronic illness, but it would need to be combined with information on complications and cause-of-death data from hospitals and civil registration systems to understand the burden of disease which each of these chronic illnesses are causing. Conversely, many cases of chronic diseases like HIV and tuberculosis—especially its drug resistant forms—are identified in tertiary care sites. Without adding this data, the primary care data would underestimate the prevalence of such diseases. This is also true for complications and deaths in many acute communicable diseases, where diagnosis occurs only at the tertiary care site.

There are many illnesses of public health importance, which just cannot be captured on survey as the sample sizes required would be too large, or because they are not picked up in self-reported surveys. Some of these, for example leprosy, are detected through special mobilization efforts at the primary care level, while others like cancers and neurological diseases require well-kept registries at the secondary and tertiary care level. Among the new indicators proposed for health systems as part of the post-2015 Sustainable Development Goals is preventable mortalities before the age of 70 (United Nations 2015). Only a nation with a robust civil registration system with reliable cause-of-death reporting would be able to measure this.

2.7 **Measuring Health Coverage: Data on Service Delivery and Organization of Services**

The most commonly collected routine health information relates to the utilization of services at facility, community, or hospital levels. When seen in context of the potential target population—that is, what proportion of all those who should have received those services, actually received it—then we have a utilization rate which, in most systems, is the data most often used to measure coverage. Two types of data, making up the numerator and denominator, respectively, are needed in order to calculate coverage or utilization rates. First, the numerator is made up of the number of patient or client encounters with the health services. This is an anonymized aggregate number, for example the number of infants under one year having received a measles vaccine, and which is typically derived from health service records. Second, the target population, for example the number of infants under one year, is making up the denominator when calculating utilization and coverage rates for measles immunization. Examples of utilization rates are 'OPD [outpatient department] visits per capita per year' and 'hospitalizations per year per 1000 population', and examples of coverage rates are 'percentage of children below 1 who have received their full immunization schedule', or 'percentage of pregnant women who have received full antenatal care as defined'.

With reference to Figure 2.3, we see that the calculation of health services coverage, which is a key feature of public health information systems and informatics, is based on both population-based data sources and health service-based data sources. This is in stark contrast to the clinical perspective on information systems, which focuses on the individual and their health records.

Health equity is one of the most important goals of public health. When we measure access or coverage, we need to do so by specific disaggregations based on sex, economic and social status, ethnic and community backgrounds, rural or urban residence, so as to measure health equity. This makes it possible to improve access to key services to more vulnerable populations. The challenge in measuring equity through calculation of health services coverage is twofold, as it is necessary to both record the services provided to each group and estimate their target population through surveys or census data. This illustrates the need for both population-based and health service-based data sources in public health information systems.

It is also possible to measure quality of care using carefully chosen data sets and indicators, to assess overall achievement. Quality has many dimensions, but the most important would be effectiveness and safety. The other dimensions of quality of care, which may be more difficult to measure, include patient comfort, satisfaction, and the dignity, privacy, and respect for an individual's rights with which care was provided.

Again such measurements cannot come from only one source. Thus, the electronic health records of a hospital would have nothing to say about social exclusion of the marginalized from care. Nor would we be able to comment on the effectiveness of primary care without hospital records, which shows us admissions for complications. Even for tracking and supporting referrals from primary care providers to specialists and vice versa, one needs a suitable supporting information system. Since for many illnesses those seeking care may consult multiple providers, even counting illness episodes and disease prevalence requires the ability to integrate information from different sources without double counting or missing critical health events. If technical and institutional means for this are not made available, effective coverage could be seriously overestimated.

2.8 **On the Nature of Population-based Information Systems and Health Services**

In section 2.7 we argued that (also) being population-based in terms of data sources and use areas are key characteristics of public health information systems. This focus on the population, or target groups, or service-user groups is in contrast to the clinical information systems perspective where the focus will typically be on the individual. Population and patient-based clinical systems are different in that they are used for different purposes and are developed and designed according to different logics. In the context of public health informatics, it is important to understand the difference between these types of systems and what population-based means in terms of system design. Here we will identify and describe two important population-based features in public health information systems: first, the use of population-based data, such as from censuses and surveys, as denominators in calculating indicators; and second, information support of population-based health services, such as antenatal care and immunization.

Population-based data, such as from censuses and estimates of target populations, make up a central component of the public health information system, as these data are used as denominators in the calculation of coverage indicators. Public health information systems have, as a rule, a strong denominator focus. These denominator data will always have a certain margin of error and will rarely be accurate. The number used for expected pregnancies in African countries will typically be calculated as four per cent of the estimated population for an area, which again will be based on annual estimates of population growth since the last census, typically carried out many years earlier. Such 'estimates of estimates' will never be accurate. These denominator data are therefore of a different type than the numerator data, which are typically the 'counts' of the services being rendered at the health facility, whether the numbers are aggregated from electronic records, paper registers, or tick sheets. While the target population denominator data in most cases will be estimates and characterized with a certain uncertainty and fuzziness, the numerator data are different in that they aim at being accurate. Of course, there are also huge data quality issues with the numerator data aggregated from the health services records. But the point here is that there are different types of systems and methodologies used to arrive at the data components of an indicator. We discuss data quality issues related to population data and their relation to complexity in Chapter 7.

We also include information support to population-based health services more generally, to be part of what we term the population-based perspective of public health information systems. Immunization and mother and child health services are population based, in that the primary aim is to reach the entire target population and not only those that are coming to the health facilities. While aiming at identifying and reaching the population unable to access particular health services, we have even greater challenges regarding open-endedness and uncertainty with population data in general. Information systems to support population-based health services will therefore also have a certain open-ended scope in its reach and design. As primary healthcare expands with increasing resources and political commitment the number of such population-based health services increases.

While highlighting the population-based aspects of public health information systems and what distinguishes these systems from typical clinical approaches, it is important to emphasize that public health information systems also include medical records and other clinical approaches. Ensuring continuity of care for tuberculosis (TB) and HIV/AIDS patients, and for other patients with chronic diseases in communities, is typically central to clinical approaches, but is also part of the PHI approach, since this is a public obligation with considerable externalities. Similarly, many aspects of district hospital management form part of both clinical and public health informatics. Clinical approaches are therefore also part of the public health informatics framework, which may be understood as approaches to extend appropriate clinical approaches; from the individual treated in the hospital, to all those requiring care in the community. The other way is also true; population-based 'serve the people' perspectives will help focus and also improve clinical approaches. It is therefore important to see population and clinically-based approaches as a continuum of mutual synergies.

2.9 **Information for Health Governance and Public Health Management: Cross-cutting Health Systems-based Analysis**

All management is essentially about the processes involved in converting available inputs to achieve the maximum possible objectives. Public health management in the usual LMIC is always a struggle to optimize health outcomes from the very limited financial, human, and material resources available. Governance concerns the challenges of making policy choices, setting priorities, deciding strategy, making resource allocation, and ensuring accountability. Every one of these actions requires more and more information, best approached through a systems framework, which seeks to understand interlinkages between the organization of service delivery, human resources, access to medical technologies, financing of healthcare, information systems, management, and governance.

With regard to human resources, the introduction of ICTs has made hitherto routine personnel management functions like payroll and salaries, postings, transfers, and promotions easier, and has also improved recruitment and skills development processes. But the real power of ICTs would be realized by going beyond this and using cross-cutting analysis to improve the efficiency and quality of service delivery. Better allocation of resources, measurement of workforce performance, and better delivery of incentives can all be facilitated by PHIs. Similarly, ICTs have demonstrated their use for the management of logistics and inventory systems that enhance access to essential drugs and diagnostics. When combined with turnover of drugs, it provides valuable information about morbidity patterns, and about utilization of services and efficiency of care. This taken in conjunction with service delivery data can be scaled to the population level. Similarly, computerization of financial information in addition to increasing the ease of accounting and auditing, when combined with the study of patterns and rates of expenditure, can provide vital information about the progress of programmes and schemes and make budgeting and financial flows more responsive to needs.

Another important dimension that has recently evoked considerable interest relates to result-based financing, or performance-based financing (Meessen *et al.* 2011), with the intent to promote certain types of provider behaviour and motivation. Result-based and performance-based financing requires information to have much higher standards of reliability and verifiability. More often than not, such payments would not only require information about the quantity of services delivered, but also considerable details about the quality of care, especially the adherence to standard treatment guidelines, and checks against irrational or excessive care provision, denial of care, or fraud of different types. Many countries are shifting to a model involving the greater role of the government in purchasing care, rather than directly providing it. Purchasing care could be typically through insurance mechanisms, or a wide variety of contracting arrangements, or through partnerships with the private sector. By necessity, today all insurance schemes are supported by HIS and there is much to learn in developing these.

There are two related information challenges here. One is collating information on out-of-pocket expenditures, which is not captured as part of routine reporting, but is becoming central to the measurement of health systems' performance in the context of universal health coverage. The second is the ability to cull aggregate information of public health importance out of the individual level insurance and other purchase-of-care arrangements. But the interoperability required between different information systems to achieve such objectives is often absent.

Health information therefore can be characterized as 'the tide that lifts all the boats', as it can help improve workforce management; access to technologies and the financing of healthcare; support better planning and implementation of all health programmes; and the better organization of service delivery. Information is also the glue that binds together all these building blocks with the leadership and governance of the health sector. Public health informatics is essentially about the generation, analysis, dissemination, and use of information required for making these decisions.

2.10 **Public Health as Never Before: 'Health in All'**

The scope of public health goes far beyond what actors in the health sector must do. To quote the Alma-Ata Declaration again: 'It includes at least: education concerning prevailing health problems and the methods of preventing and controlling them; promotion of food supply and proper nutrition; an adequate supply of safe water and basic sanitation; maternal and child healthcare, including family planning; immunisation against the major infectious diseases; prevention and control of locally endemic diseases; appropriate treatment of common diseases and injuries; and provision of essential drugs. It also involves, in addition to the health sector, all related sectors and aspects of national and community development, in particular agriculture, animal husbandry, food, industry, education, housing, public works, communications and other sectors; and demands the coordinated efforts of all those sectors' (WHO 1978, Declaration VII). The latter is now referred as the 'Health in All' policies.

Cross-sector health impact assessment of all policies is increasingly being recognized as essential—even indispensable. For example, the rise in food prices, or the enforcement of laws against air pollution, or introduction of road safety measures or increasing duties on tobacco products and alcohol, could each have an immediate influence on health outcomes. As every sector gets to grips with using digital platforms, the possibilities of studying and correlating trends in morbidity with policy changes and changes in the determinants of disease become immense. Finland is an acknowledged leader in this area. But such work has barely begun in most LMICs.

Knowledge of the relationship between the social and environmental determinants of health and morbidity trends can catalyse policy change, as well as influence individual lifestyles and health-related practices. Knowledge on the link between cancer and tobacco use, or rise of admissions for acute respiratory illness during peaks of urban air pollution have been critical for driving control measures that address these determinants. Many disease–environment links require a much higher quality of health records. For example, the incidence of mesothelioma, a fatal form of lung cancer that occurs almost always due to exposure to asbestosis, is seriously underestimated in most LMICs, simply because there are no cancer registries or that the existing registries capture only a fraction of the desired health events and with insufficient quality.

It is also essential to recognize that access to such information should not be limited to policy makers, but must be available on the public domain. It is the weight of public opinion that, more often than not, drives pro-health policy changes. The forces that shape policy are many. In most contexts, the interests of industry and politically powerful elite would predominate, unless confronted with evidence which points to the impact on health and argues it from an equity perspective. And this not only needs information, but a transparency on how this information is collected, aggregated, and interpreted.

One principle of 'health for all', stated with great brevity and precision in the Alma-Ata Declaration is: 'The people have the right and duty to participate individually and collectively in the planning and implementation of their healthcare' (WHO 1978, Declaration IV). There are many reasons for providing communities a greater role, including strengthening democratic participation and accountability of public health systems. Communities can and do play a valuable role in priority setting and in choice of strategies, especially as regards access to services. Accessible, relevant health information can empower communities to participate much more effectively at the local level.

Health informatics has too often seen itself as only the tool of the provider and the individual patient. But public health informatics needs to re-discover the meaning of the word *public*, not only as an object of study but also as one of its primary subjects, that is, as one of main users of health information.

2.11 **The Interface with Clinical Informatics**

Whereas clinical informatics can exist without public health informatics, in our understanding public health informatics incorporates the entire field of clinical informatics, and far beyond. Also, it does not perceive clinical informatics as some form of first phase or foundational premise on which the rest of the edifice of PHI is erected. In fact, in most national contexts the institutional capacity to build public health informatics on a substrate of electronic health records is not currently present, and will take time to develop. Furthermore, the extensive use of clinical electronic health records is by itself no assurance that the information needs of public health can be culled out of it. Specific technical and institutional efforts, which currently are poorly developed, are required to do so.

Having said that, we highlight five reasons why public health informatics must be developed as a continuum with clinical informatics.

2.11.1 **For creating a continuum between clinical and population-based approaches**

Clinical approaches, ranging from the running of district hospitals to the provision of curative services in the community and the running of HIV/AIDS and TB programmes, are all part of the public health approach. To provide information support to these clinically oriented health services and programmes are therefore well within the scope of public health informatics, which may be understood as extending appropriate clinical approaches from the hospital into the community. It is therefore important to see population-based and clinically-based approaches as a continuum.

2.11.2 **For ease of recording**

Most data elements related to delivery or utilization of services are records of specific clinical encounters. Most primary providers do not currently use electronic health records for recording the encounter, but record these on paper and report them as aggregate numbers, often supported by a digital platform. Digitization saves the care provider of additional burden of work in aggregation and reporting and enables analysis of his or her own achievements. But to be viable, digital primary records must substitute, and not add to manual recording.

2.11.3 **For continuity of care**

Organization of primary healthcare requires integrated, functional, and mutually supportive referral systems, leading to the progressive improvement in healthcare for all, and giving priority to those most in need. Much of the effectiveness and credibility of primary care depends on building good information flows across healthcare providers, making it important to create electronic health records which primary providers find convenient to use, and which are visible to secondary and tertiary care providers, and vice versa. Such to and from referral linkages are also essential across public and private providers, and between specialist consultations.

2.11.4 **For assuring access to care**

There is an ethical obligation to ensure that no person is denied access to an adequate quality of healthcare, irrespective of their ability to pay for it. In many nations this is a legal right, not merely an ethical one, representing a fundamental human right guaranteed by the constitution. The reality is that this objective is quite far off for most LMICs, but constitutes a fundamental objective to strive for. And further access is seen to have been achieved or to be coverage effective, only when there is evidence of good quality of care. The clinical case record makes both the access to care and the quality of care provided to individuals more transparent and verifiable, and therefore also the subgroup or population that we are concerned about.

2.11.5 **For ensuring patient rights and autonomy in clinical care**

In the name of public priorities, the state can encroach on civil liberties of individuals. For example, the state has a duty to ensure that every tuberculosis patient completes his or treatment, but on the other hand, the fact that a person has tuberculosis is confidential that only the patient has the right to reveal. The performance of the state duty towards protecting privacy, confidentiality, dignity, and the choice of the individual over his or her own body and decisions made about it, requires both design features, organization of work flows, and governance and regulatory features. The state's duty to protect public health could often pull in opposing directions with implications for the interface between public health and clinical informatics. Whereas clinical information and records are essential, for most public purposes this data would be available only in its PHI form, which is as anonymized and aggregated.

All this leads to one inescapable conclusion—that the emerging discipline of PHI must be an amalgam of population-based information and individual health records. Here the needs of individuals seeking and providing care, and the needs of communities and governments to ensure the attainment of the highest level of health for the population are seamlessly integrated into a single health information architecture.

2.12 **Evolution and Path Dependence of Public Health Informatics**

In the early 1990s, across most nations, health information systems began to develop around the new 'digital' or 'electronic' ICTs. The health systems context in which this happened influenced what information was first computerized, what uses it was put to, and perceptions regarding the purpose of HIS and how it could lead to improved health outcomes. Many problems and limitations, as well as strengths of the currently available system, are better understood in the historical context of its evolution, which we broadly categorize into three main paths.

2.12.1 **Origins in monitoring vertical programmes and health sector reforms**

The most common evolutionary path for HIS, quite typical of India, Bangladesh, and most African nations, is where it has developed as a key component of the ongoing health sector reforms. The context for these reforms was the structural adjustment programmes largely guided by the World Bank and international aid agencies such as the United States Agency for International Development (USAID) and the Department for International Development (DFID). Such programmes tended to focus on vertical healthcare interventions which sought to bring greater visibility to the effectiveness of their aid. Furthermore, under structural adjustment, governments were required to be very selective about public health interventions, leaving the rest of the sector subject to market forces. This led to a focus on reproductive health, immunization, fertility control, and on some major communicable diseases like tuberculosis, malaria, leprosy, and HIV. It was recognized in these reform efforts that effective monitoring and supervision were important, and this meant that every donor had to provide the programme management for the activities they were funding. Since there were different donors and different interventions, it was simpler for each to build HISs that were dedicated and designed to monitor the specific programme that they were funding.

As a result, most LMICs were saddled with multiple vertically oriented HIS for particular health programmes with limited interoperability. Typically these systems dealt with large amounts of aggregate numbers (and typically not as indicators) all flowing upward to the central monitoring office. There were some exceptions, such as the tuberculosis control programmes, which included a good hierarchy of indicators in their HIS. There were rarely linkages with civil registration of vital events, or with financing, supplies, or human resources management systems. In recent years, various governments have initiated efforts to make primary record entry name-based instead of the aggregate number-based, which, it is assumed, (wrongly, we will argue) will help deal with the problem of overreporting.

There have been various national efforts recently to study and improve issues of data quality, and the increasing use of targets. One common observation is that in a reprimand culture there are perverse incentives that work against honest reporting, leading to data quality challenges. Another equally important reason is that when data is not converted into indicators using suitable denominators, it is almost worthless for informing action. In addition, very often there are mismatches between what is collected as data and what is needed for indicators. Furthermore, there are problems of data definitions and rules of when to collect and whom to report to, which are not well understood by those collecting and reporting data. Often the same event is recorded from multiple sites and are therefore overcounted, or the same event is reported into multiple systems causing poor data quality and excessive burden on the staff. When there are many problems in data collection, and are not addressed in design, computerization only helps to automate existing inefficiencies, making them more difficult to rectify in future. Poor data quality undermines use of information, an aspect that we discuss in detail in Chapter 3.

2.12.2 Origins in building primary care systems

In a few LMICs, and in some most developed nations, the nature of care was comprehensive to begin with, and despite pressures or because of the lack of external funding, they never went for selective care, as for example, Brazil and Thailand. To some extent Sri Lanka and South Africa are also good examples of this, though in later years South Africa was also to have a fair share of vertical programmes. These systems are simple, but robust, and there is clarity on what is required. Thailand's system is a good example of this. The Health Centre Information Service of its Ministry of Public Health has over 80 per cent of the facilities reporting on administrative and clinical information. They are used for reimbursement to hospitals, for facility activity monitoring, and for measurement and evaluation. They are also used to support clinical work mainly through medical record keeping. There are two minimal data sets that every facility reports on: the 'Standard Data Set for Health Insurance', which is a 12-file data set for hospitals, including outpatient and inpatient information by costs, and by diagnosis and procedure. Its main aim is to support hospital reimbursement, but as collateral, other public health data also becomes available. The second minimum data set is for primary care units, which is an 18-file data set, providing outpatient data by diagnosis, and information on preventive and promotive health activities. While reporting on these two data sets is obligatory, which system to use is not. Standards to ensure interoperability across multiple systems have been declared, including semantic (covering disease diagnosis, national drugs codes, and medical terminologies), syntactic (HL7 messaging standards, HL7, CDA (clinical document architecture)), and for privacy and confidentiality (Boonchai 2014). In Thailand, there are fewer systems in operation and therefore the problem of multiple systems operating in silos is not so acute. This also contributes to greater use of information for financial management, HR management, and on-facility performance.

2.12.3 **Origins in insurance-based systems—mainly in developed nations**

All insurance systems have adopted information technology platforms, and are deployed in empanelled hospitals for the processing of claims. At present in LMICs, very little use is made of information that flows from the claims settlement process even though millions of claims are processed. Taken together, this reflects population-based data of a different type. Its use even for monitoring is very low. It is however important to note that there is a health informatics that originates in electronic health records, and then extracts public health information from it as collateral—more of an afterthought than the intention.

In the United States, data that is present is largely the property of private insurance companies or health management organizations linked to privately owned and managed health information exchanges (HIEs) which facilitate communication between organizations. The main data source is health records used in processing insurance claims. Over the years, an enormous database of such records has become available, representing 'big data' typically used for fraud detection, for data analytics supporting the pharmaceutical industry, and in identifying opportunities for cost savings, and so on. There is relatively limited use in understanding the health of a population defined by geography or by a social group, which can strengthen public health surveillance activities and research.

In nations with tax-financed universal public insurance like the United Kingdom, Canada, Australia, and New Zealand, the development of health records to support both primary and hospital care was given emphasis but was accompanied by parallel developments of PHIs. Given the health systems context where the vast majority of health encounters are paid for by public financing and/or delivered by public facilities, PHI arose by extracting information from the case records. In United Kingdom, there are four organizations engaged in mining electronic health records, in order to cull aggregate population-based data: the Health and Social Care Information Centre (HSCIC, a replacement of the old National Health Service (NHS) Information Centre) which is a management tool of the NHS; the Clinical Practice Research Data Link (CPRD), mainly a primary healthcare research support tool; the Clinical Commissioning Groups (CCG), part of the contracting process; and, Public Health England (PHE), which deals with PHI. PHE collects vast amounts of data from GP surgeries, hospitals, and NHS laboratories as part of its health surveillance and protection activities, and links this data to data sets such as Hospital Episode Statistics, the Office of National Statistics mortality data, and those generated by activities such as the genomic sequencing of infectious disease agents (House of Parliament UK 2014).

This section has contextualized the evolution of PHIs within a historical perspective. This has helped to identify the trajectories of growth, and the challenges of the disconnect between clinical/individual information and aggregate data, or statistics.

This leads us to the next section where certain guiding principles are identified for PHIs.

2.13 Establishing Principles of Design for the 'Expanded PHI' Approach for Low and Middle-Income Countries

After situating PHI within an informatics and public health perspective in Chapters 1 and 2, respectively, we now develop the argument for what we will term (for the lack of a better alternative) an 'Expanded PHI' approach in LMICs, to guide both academics and practice. We present five such broad design principles that at a meta-level can help guide.

1. A multidisciplinary and systems approach to its study
2. Building open architectures, not stand-alone systems
3. Multidisciplinary certainly, but with public health at its core
4. Contextualization
5. Plurality of methods for its development with action research at the core

2.13.1 Multidisciplinary and systems-based approaches

Arguably, the evolution of both approaches has each been characterized by a narrow focus. While in the rich countries, the field of health informatics— informed primarily by computers, information, and cognitive sciences—has dominated, leading to an individual and patient-based focus, in LMICs, the focus has been on population-based systems for monitoring selective primary healthcare interventions. There has been largely an absence of a guiding academic approach to support this evolution in LMICs. The 'Expanded PHI' approach we argue for, needs to design and develop systems that transcend both, enabling an individual focus which can be rolled up to the population level, and also population-based systems which lend themselves to being rolled back to individual persons, events, or locations. The core of this is to understand information needs at different levels of use, with the ability to cater for each at the desired level of granularity, and yet retain a primary perspective of understanding the implications on population health. This then necessarily requires a multiplicity of perspectives to be incorporated, including informatics, information sciences, public health, development studies, implementation research, institutional theory, and various others. This multiplicity will need to be adopted both in the practice of designing and implementing systems for public health, and also in supporting academic studies of PHI.

More than four decades of research in information systems globally has helped us learn that 'aeroplanes don't fly, airlines do'. This implies that technology (in this case, the aeroplane) cannot bring change by itself, but needs to be supported by an integrated and heterogeneous network comprising of multiple institutions (such as ticketing, air traffic control, baggage services), infrastructure (baggage belts, runways, airport buses, ticketing software), people, procedures, and practices which guide the working of these different institutions. Furthermore, these different and heterogeneous actors (human and non-human) need to be seamlessly inter-connected with each other. A break in any part of the network has implications which propagate to the whole. These networked linkages are most evident in PHIs in LMICs, as there are various different non-human actors such as diseases, infrastructure, geography, technology, and human actors such as government staff, health workers, donors, technology vendors, healthcare organizations, and others. All these need to be aligned effectively in heterogeneous networks for systems to be optimally designed and used.

This learning has significant implications on models and concepts used to study PHIs, and to build the practice of how systems (or architectures) are designed, built, and sustained over time. Various social science and technology approaches have been developed in information systems, for example, theories from science and technology studies, such as Actor–Network and Information Infrastructure. These theories have been evolved to inform systems research and practice, and later applied to HIS work in both developed and developing country settings. An academic approach to Expanded PHIs in LMICs would need to be grounded in such social science approaches, within the context and realities of LMICs, to develop relevant knowledge that could inform practice.

Implementation is a crucial component of PHIs, and going beyond technology design, implementation efforts would need to be informed by fields such as sociology, social work, anthropology, history, and organizational behaviour and institutional analysis.

In summary, we argue for the Expanded PHI approach in LMICs to be necessarily multidisciplinary in design, to contribute to understanding the multifaceted and socio-technical nature of the phenomenon.

2.13.2 Building open architectures—not stand-alone systems

Adopting a plurality of approaches and perspectives must necessarily have at its core the need to understand how systems can speak to each other, both technically and institutionally. The single biggest identified challenge to strengthening HIS has been of fragmentation, which impedes development of the more holistic understandings of health systems, PHI challenges, and solutions. For example, the immunization manager at a district does not only need data on vaccines coverage, as is normally the case, but also requires data on other services offered to the catchment population, and on cold chain functioning, supply chain logistics, and human resources availability, as well as the incidence of vaccine-preventable diseases and the possible adverse effects of immunization. Furthermore, it is important to understand who are the children at risk, the reasons why, and the addresses of the children, so that appropriate care can be provided. The paradox is that most of this information is already available on different digitized platforms, but cross-cutting analysis is not possible because each of these is in a silo with limited ability to communicate with each other.

Often, there are different information systems being used: one for the individual child receiving immunization, and the other for aggregate reporting from the catchment population. In such a context, the individual systems should have the ability to roll up to the catchment population. Similarly, aggregated systems should allow the manager to drill down to identify the particular child at risk. This would allow for controlling the burden of data collection, building greater data integrity, and enabling more accurate data analysis to strengthen evidence-based action. Such 'speaking of systems to each other' must by necessity be supported by a more holistic and health systems-based understanding.

The reasons for current fragmentation are many, and all of these together constrain efforts at health systems strengthening. These include the dominance of vertical programmes, multiplicity of donors and their interventions, and stand-alone departments defending their particular turfs. More than three decades of research into these challenges has developed an understanding for the need of an architecture-based approach, which has at its heart a design of systems speaking to each other, both technically and institutionally (Braa and

Sahay 2012). Such architectures necessarily needs to be 'open' (software and standards) to enable this inter-system linking, and this forms the core of the Expanded PHI approach.

We discuss in Chapter 4 why open architecture is not just a technical problem, but it also has significant institutional implications such as changing systems of procurement which are currently geared towards proprietary solutions, and the development of human resources, skills, and mind-sets towards these inter-connected systems. Both academics and practice, which have historically focused on multiple, parallel, silo-based systems, need to be fundamentally changed to address this fragmentation problem, especially with regard to the future challenges of universal health coverage and improved civil registration and vital statistics systems, which we take up in Chapter 8.

2.13.3 Multidisciplinary—certainly, but with public health at its core

The academic field of health informatics has found it difficult to find a stable home in universities, because its underlying multidisciplinarity is both a strength and weakness. In many sites of its development as a discipline, the field has been largely dominated by clinicians and people from informatics, reflecting a strong bias towards technical and clinical systems at the expense of a public health focus. This is a problem, especially for LMICs, where one of the urgent needs of the system is the support required for health systems management. The public health and programme logic underlying these systems is often conspicuous by its absence, and even large-scale systems tend to be developed by technical staff with limited public health inputs. This lack has time and again contributed to 'design-reality' gaps (Heeks 2002) and systems failures.

The Expanded PHI approach in LMICs needs by necessity to have public health and principles of information systems at its core, to ensure that the development of these systems is driven by health system needs and not the interests and perceptions of the technologists and donors. Given the multiplicity of the actors involved, and their competing interests and logics, inputs from political science are important to understand governance challenges arising from the needs to address a multiplicity of interests and how they may be tackled.

2.13.4 Contextualization

Context matters and this insight has been a fundamental learning in information systems research for both developed and developing countries. Simply understood, context refers to pre-existing conditions of history, culture, politics, institutions, capacities, and infrastructure. These existing conditions have the power to influence and shape the dynamics around design, development, and implementation of HIS solutions. However, the influences are not unidirectional, and new technologies hold the potential of bringing about changes in the existing context, although often taking place over years, rather than months. Developing deep and conceptual understandings of the context, and the nature of its mutual (shaping and shaped) influences with technology initiatives should be a key endeavour to Expanded PHI approaches.

2.13.5 Plurality of methods for development with action research at the core

While the principles or design we have just identified are important to define the ontology of knowledge, or the nature of understanding the subject under study, the other related question is of epistemology, concerning how to try and access that knowledge. The health informatics and informatics traditions of North America are typically positivist; geared towards formulating hypotheses, testing them in controlled environments, and building models for statistical generalizability.

We argue to shift this emphasis in at least three ways.

The first is towards the adoption of a more interpretivist approach that emphasizes the subjectivities of the different actors involved, and focuses on understanding how processes of inter-subjectivity are generated. This then necessarily involves building an understanding of different subjective meanings that people attribute, and try to relate them to their respective contexts to understand the why behind those meanings. Such an approach is arguably more in line with our broadly social-scientific mode of inquiry being advocated here.

The second is the need to build on the more effective 'realistic evaluation' methods. Such an evaluation approach does not merely ask, 'Does this system work'? but says, 'to what extent does this system work, and in what circumstances, why, and for whose benefit'? Realist evaluation approaches will help to fill the gap of the very limited evaluation efforts typically accompanying health informatics efforts in LMICs. It contextualizes the evaluation analysis to the actors, interests, and motives they bring to the table. Realist evaluation makes explicit the often implicit theories of change—how better information systems are expected to lead to better health outcomes—and uses these to study the relationship of the context, the intervention, and the outcomes.

The third is to develop and use more effective action research methods, since our focus is not only to study, but to also build better technologies to strengthen health systems. This necessarily requires an approach that is action oriented, and built on collaboration between the researcher and those having an interest in the system being developed. It involves development of prototypes in multiple contexts for multiple needs, and then learning and generalizing from these. However, this approach also raises the big challenge of 'too much action, too little research'. The experiences of the two-decade long and ongoing University of Oslo HISP (Health Information Systems Programme) action research programme is a case study that provides a rich repository of learning and inspiration for building on and enlarging this Expanded PHI approach.

2.14 **Conclusions**

In Chapters 1 and 2, building on the historical sketches of the trends in informatics and health informatics, and understanding their implications for academics and practice, we have tried to articulate some underlying design principles for what we have tentatively termed an 'Expanded PHI approach'.

If the first of these chapters is a strong caution against linking informatics too closely to computerization as technology, the second is against confusing the clinical health concerns with those of public health. Both chapters highlight that even where the objectives addressed are explicitly public health related and the systems context is acknowledged, the lack of alternative theoretical approaches to the development of this discipline leads to a widespread proliferation of initiatives to apply ICTs in LMICs with suboptimal results, and the development of PHIs is a stunted, faltering growth, nowhere living up to the huge expectations. The future promises more of such efforts, involving more complex and resource intensive systems. To help guide these endeavours, there is thus an urgent need to build a strong academic and practice basis to adopt and build upon the 'Expanded PHI approach', one that learns from historical developments in informatics and health, but is deeply grounded in the local realities and priorities.

This book is a step in this direction.

2.15 **References**

Boonchai, K. (2014). Thailand Primary Health Care Information Systems [Online]. Available at: http://www.whofic-apn.com/pdf_files/4th_19_11p.pdf [Accessed: 10 October 2014].

Braa, J. and Sahay, S. (2012). *Integrated Health Information Architecture: Power to the Users: Design, Development and Use*. Matrix Publishers, New Delhi, India.

Health Metrics Network (2008). *Health Metrics Network, Framework and Standards for the Development of Country Health Information Systems*. World Health Organization. Available at: http://apps.who.int/iris/bitstream/10665/43872/1/9789241595940_eng.pdf [Accessed: 01 February 2016].

Heeks, R. (2002). Information systems and developing countries: failure, success, and local improvisations. *The Information Society*, **18**, 101–12.

House of Parliament UK (2014). Big Data and Public Health, POSTnote, Parliamentary Office of Science & Technology, No.474.

Meessen, B., Soucat, A., and Sekabaraga, C. (2011). Performance-based financing: just a donor fad or a catalyst towards comprehensive health-care reform?. *Bulletin of the World Health Organization*, **89**(2), 153–6.

United Nations (2015). Transforming our world: the 2030 Agenda for Sustainable Development. Post-2015 process. [Online]. Available at: https://sustainabledevelopment.un.org/post2015/transformingourworld [Last accessed: 1 October 2015].

WHO (1978). Declaration of Alma-Ata, International Conference on Primary Health Care. Alma-Ata, USSR, 6–12 September 1978. Available at: http://www.who.int/publications/almaata_declaration_en.pdf [Last accessed: 1 October 2015].

WHO (2008). Primary health care—now more than ever. *World Health Report*, World Health Organization, p. 55.

WHO (2007). Everybody's business: strengthening health systems to improve health outcomes. WHO's Framework for Action, Geneva, p. 3

Winslow, C.E.A. (1920). The untilled fields of public health. *Science*, **51**(1306), 23–33, cited in http://www.lib.berkeley.edu/PUBL/whatisph.html [Accessed: 30 June 2015]

Chapter 3

The 'Information-Use Problematic' in Health Information Systems

The information you *have* is not the information you *want*
The information you *want* is not the information you *need*
The information you *need* is not easy to *obtain*
The information you *obtain* is not worth the costs *you pay* for it.

Finagle's Laws of (Public Health) Information

3.1 The 'Use of Information' Problematic in General

Using information is a continuing and perplexing problem which permeates all organizations, not just those concerning health. This problem has been studied in depth by researchers in organization studies and information systems, under various labels of information for decision-making, evidence-based decisions, decision support systems, expert systems, and others. An underlying assumption in these efforts is the underlying rational and common sense view that if information is provided, the 'decision maker' will make an informed choice, which will maximize efficiency and financial returns. This comes largely from the assumptions of an 'economic man' from economics, drawing upon universal principles of rationality and efficiency related to profit maximization. Over the years, these assumptions have largely been debunked. The conditions the economists stipulate for their models of 'all other things being constant' do not hold in real life when there are human beings and organizations involved, and their interests are central in how decisions are made. Various other motives for taking decisions have been identified, other than that of rationality. For example, it has now been publicly acknowledged that the US and UK governments went ahead with the decision to go to war in Iraq based on flawed intelligence and without UN security council approval. The South African government long resisted the evidence that HIV leads to AIDS, to make their argument that the disease was largely a Western conspiracy. Sahay and Walsham (1996) showed that while GIS models were developed to determine optimal locations for digging wells based on scientific principles in India, in reality decisions based on political preferences for pleasing con-stituencies were made. The resource dependency perspective proponents have emphatically argued that decisions are made to favour certain alliances where there are resource dependencies to be nurtured. In her seminal book *Plans and Situated Actions* Lucy Suchman (1987) argued that the reasons why people make choices are a product of their cultural environment, and as a result these choices vary according to situational context. Sahay (1997) has described how the (lack of) use of maps in India is culturally bound, and even senior GIS researchers would prefer to ask people for directions rather than consult a map.

We argue that this learning on theories of decision-making is indeed very rel-evant in the public health sector in low and middle-income countries (LMICs) when we discuss 'use of information' or 'information for action', because it underlies similar rationalistic assumptions that if health programme managers are provided relevant information, they will take action, and health improve-ments will ensue. Many of us have thus been engaged in designing systems to ensure appropriate information can be made available to managers, and others have studied to see if managers actually use this information. Results have been largely negative, with broad conclusions made that 'there is little or no use of information being made' and new solutions are searched for in terms of pro-viding faster information, or on mobile devices to ensure that the 'information reaches the decision maker on the fingertips'.

Availability of information is a necessary, but not a sufficient condition to ensure effective usage. And conditions of sufficiency come or are withheld through reasons of politics, resource dependency, groupthink, and various others. So our perennial quest of seeing or enabling enhanced information use by providing more actionable information may be a case of searching for *a needle which is not in the haystack*! In this chapter, we will like to flip the information use problem on its head. Rather than try to identify why informa-tion is not being used, as many studies have already done previously, we will focus on the question of what are the characteristics of health systems where we see information is broadly valued and viewed as a resource to strengthen the system. In other words, we seek to understand what these conditions of sufficiency are, and how this can be enabled, with a socio-technical rather than solely technological focus. Arguably, this has implications for the design of information systems and sets up the need for what we are tentatively calling an Expanded PHI approach.

3.1.1 Use of information in health

The use of health information presents a contemporary problematic, which many stakeholders, including ministries, donors, state- and district-level managers, and global agencies are constantly trying to address, but often with limited results. This problematic represents a paradox, where data overload impedes relevant information use; to solve this, more information technology (IT) systems are deployed creating more data, which further confounds information use. Finagle's laws on information may be humorous, but they are insightful in understanding this paradox.

IT solutions are often not sensitively designed to the context, ending up providing lots of data which does not stimulate action, and could even on occasions do the reverse. Relevant information remains buried in the mass of data collection, and in reaching this stage of data flow, the energy to use it is dissipated. Why is this the case, and what can be done about it? These are the issues that this chapter seeks to address. Technology and information are not ends in themselves, but only means to better decisions in policy design, health planning, management, monitoring, and the evaluation of programmes and services (Lippeveld *et al.* 2000).

While there is much more data in flow than what existed before, this statement by Chambers of more than three decades ago is as true now as it was then—or even more so.

> Much of the material remains unprocessed … or
> If processed, unanalysed … or
> If analysed, not read … Or
> If read, not used or acted upon
> Only a miniscule proportion of the findings affect policy, and they are usually a few simple totals
>
> (Chambers 1983).

Despite the massive advances in computerization and IT enabling health information systems, the analysis and use of information in decision-making remains limited. We begin with this problematic, because it is a powerful illustration of the challenges that public health informatics is facing. The rationale for the introduction of IT in healthcare rests on the premise that the effectiveness and efficiency of health sector performance would greatly increase with the availability of relevant information. And yet when all the technical hurdles are apparently crossed and the information made available, it not only fails to show measurable improvements in health sector performance, even its use remains very limited.

We classify broadly the reasons and pathways for suboptimal use of information into five sets. One relates to the failure of IT system design to meet and match the needs, and failing to differentiate between wants and needs. The second relates to data quality. Most programme managers and policy makers fail to use information from the systems that they have built up with such great costs and efforts, due to a perceived lack of reliable data. But then the use of data is, as we shall see, is one of the most important determinants of data quality. Thus a vicious cycle is set up, where poor use of information leads to poor data quality, which justifies poor use of data—a cycle which is not easy to break out from. A third set of reasons relates to the capacity to use information at both the institutional and individual levels. Institutional capacity relates to the skill mix needed, but part of it is also about the work processes in place for enabling the use of information, and above all a culture where information use is valued organizationally. At the individual level, health staff do not often possess the necessary incentive to use information, as they see the associated work to not be of value. Fourth, there are reasons that do not relate to information at all, but to the structure and function of the health system itself, and to the processes of governance. Finally, there are often political reasons which deter information use as it may represent the uncomfortable truth of the 'reality' becoming visible through use.

This categorization is only for convenience in discussion and to provide analytical sharpness. In real life, these reasons are intimately intertwined, and come mixed with varying emphasis in different contexts. Similarly, there is no one way of overcoming these constraints. There are many ways forward. But the contention of this book is that underlying these many ways forward—as expressed in the case studies—are some essential principles, which if internalized can be more broadly applied across situations. We start with an extended case study example from Odisha, a state in India, to frame this problematic of information use (Case Study 3.1).

3.1.2 Analysing the case: Understanding information needs and systems design

We see in this case study some of the classical health information systems' design problems. The first and most obvious observation is that many systems are designed to enable central monitoring, without adequate features for enabling local use. For the local provider, entering data into the system is just another chore in addition to all her pre-existing tasks, which in any case did not become simpler, and resulting in a considerably increased workload with no benefit whatsoever. There was no need for all data collected at the village level (including names of pregnant women) to be made available in the national portal. Health facilities that had use of this data were increasingly distanced from it, when the reverse should have been the case.

There is a similar lack of functionality in the IT design for mid-level managers; in this case the district administrator and manager. Indeed, and on the contrary, there is every risk of losing existing capacity. In times of manual

(continued on page 54)

Case Study 3.1 Information Use Problem is a Product of the Health Systems: Odisha, India

Odisha is one of the states of India which lies along its eastern coast with a population of over 30 million. Most development indicators show the eastern, coastal, and largely agricultural districts of this state as doing relatively better, while the remaining districts, made up of high proportions of tribal people, have some of the poorest indicators for the entire nation. For this reason, Odisha has always attracted development aid, and the health management systems that came along with it date back to the mid-1990s.

Odisha, like all Indian states, has a four-tier public healthcare system, while the medical college hospital is at the apex and provides tertiary care. A district has about a one- to two-million population and is divided into 7 to 10 blocks with about 100,000 to 200,000 population in each—and there is a 100- to 500-bed secondary care hospital at the district level and a 10- to 30-bed hospital in each block. Primary care is provided by a network of primary health centres, each of which is led by a medical officer and caters to a 20,000 to 30,000 population. Under this primary healthcare (PHC) are four to six health subcentres managed by a nurse and a paramedical worker, providing outreach services for a 3000 to 5000 population.

When reforms began at the all-India level in 2005 under the National Rural Health Mission, Odisha was one of the states that responded eagerly to implement them to rectify their largely non-functional systems. The reforms in information systems could be discussed as happening over three phases: the first phase was in 2007–2009, representing the system redesign; the second phase was in 2010–2012, concerning the implementation of the redesigned systems; and the third phase, which is currently ongoing, represents a consolidation and integration of systems.

The first phase of system redesign involved a reduction from over 2700 data elements to a more limited three sets: about 70 data elements for the health subcentre; about 150 for the primary health centre; and about 250 for the block and district hospital. Much of the earlier excess of data elements was due to disaggregated data elements—usually by gender, age, and caste—though these were almost impossible to report on, since aggregation from the primary recording registers was still manual. Many data elements had been included at the insistence of programme divisions who felt it was important to make data elements related to their programme more visible by virtue of their appearing more on the monitoring form, even though they often had limited value for programme management. Considerable negotiations took place to effect these reductions, assisted by evidence that most data elements were reported as zeros, or were not usable, or should be collected through surveys rather than routinely. Another key reform was the setting up of a central data repository in the form of national HMIS portal to which districts were to report their aggregate data. In this phase of reforms, the message of decentralization in health systems was strong, which provided an enabling environment to also decentralize the health information systems. Thus, the policy requirement was that whereas all districts report on the national HMIS portal on a common data set and format, they could have their own systems for generating this district-level data, as each felt necessary.

The third key reform of this first phase was the putting in place of a full-time data entry operator along with the necessary hardware in every district, and training them on the new forms and skills for data entry. All these changes were organized and led at the national level by the National Rural Health Mission (NRHM) leadership, and subsequently implemented across all states. This mandate was left up to the districts to comply with, while intra-district data collection was left to the discretion of the state mission.

Results were quite dramatic with aggregate district-level data being available for the first time at district, state, and national levels. Use of information lagged behind, and was widely attributed to the unreliability of data due to false reporting. The solutions proposed to address this problem called for more granularity; firstly, facility as the unit of reporting, and then subsequently the individual names.

The second phase of reforms began in 2010. There was a new government in power now, though under the same political leadership, which provided for continuity with the earlier policies. But now the emphasis on district planning and decentralization was seriously underplayed. To improve quality of reporting, the federal government required all states to shift to facility-based reporting directly onto the national web portal. This increased the number of reporting units in Odisha from about 30 districts to over 3000 facilities—a shift that the state was in no position to undertake immediately. Also by now Odisha had in place for use a district-level system—the District Health Information Software 2 (DHIS 2), which allowed functionalities of district and subdistrict analysis. The state had moved to facility-based reporting on DHIS 2, and resisted pressures from the national HMIS team, to abandon this for direct facility reporting onto the national portal, with the argument that the latter had weak analytical capabilities. There was then a prolonged process of negotiation between central and state governments around data quality issues, where the centre attributed the problem to the state's use of DHIS 2, in preference to direct entry into the national web portal.

The solution of the division managing health informations systems at the national level to address quality issues in this second phase was that there should be only one version of the truth, which would be verified, authenticated, and officially released by the national HMIS division, and that multiple systems were confusing. And that there was no need to have district analytic capacities since an advanced statistical package (SAS) would be accessible through the national portal that would enable such analysis, and further that the centre would generate reports for statistical outliers and point these out to states, so as to improve data quality. And that if one had facility-based reporting, false reporting could be spotted and facility performance better monitored. This, in the view of almost everyone at the national and state leaderships, was the main purpose of the information system—to strengthen accountability and make monitoring more efficient.

The state government, with strong technical advice from the National Health System Resource Centre (NHSRC), a think tank providing technical advice to the Ministry of Health at the central and state levels, which in turn had a technical partnership with HISP India, a local non-governmental organization (NGO) providing support for DHIS 2, emphasized a different understanding of quality. This was centred on snags in the processes of data collection and reporting, and in this understanding wilful false reporting was not the central issue or the main contributory factor to poor data quality. Odisha had already some level of use of information anyway, and encouraged by this, they placed emphasis on feedback forms and special sessions called 'conversations over data' to promote further data use. Such conversations helped understand the data in context, trace the source of data errors, and simultaneously helped identify programme gaps. Work on enhancing greater functionalities for local district-level use of data in DHIS 2 was also expedited, and DHIS 2 evolved further with this pressure. Taken together, all this strengthened the state and district leadership's empathy with the need for decentralization, despite the changing ideological climate at the centre.

The quality improvement measures that both the state and centre agreed on in this phase were the standardization of data and indicator definitions, and various rounds of training. The discussion on all other aspects dragged on for over an year and finally met a temporary resolution when it was agreed that the data could be entered into DHIS 2 for each facility, and from there exported into a pre-coded excel sheet, to be uploaded into the national portal. The state could then proceed with its understanding of decentralized HMIS development and yet comply with central requirements. One reason why the centre now agreed to this was that the problems of data quality had not gone away with facility-based reporting in other states, but rather, they had enlarged. The centre's solution for the persistence of the problem was to go the next level of granularity—and start another system for name-based tracking of pregnant women and infants for immunization. Since this name-based system started up independently of the current HMIS, the pressure of online reporting onto the national portal could no longer be sustained in a state which was now making far more effective use of its data at the local level. The national portal in that phase still had limited features to enable district-level use of information (it took until 2013 to develop some level of district-level analysis), while the DHIS 2 analysis features had advanced, including GIS, which the state took full advantage off. Also DHIS 2 was fast becoming a global standard. None of the name-based tracking system data, despite its large volumes, was utilized in the generation of any health indicator; nor did the increased granularity give it any greater reliability as a data source. Odisha had a relatively better use of its HMIS data, but this was based largely on the fact that they had built up a system of interpreting data at participatory review meetings and had an information system that could support such use. This was the level at which the debate stabilized in 2014, when a new government came to power at the centre.

The third phase, in a sense, began with the 12th five-year plan in 2012, but came to be implemented only under the new government. In this phase, the state continued to consolidate all its data into DHIS 2, and started to focus on strengthening analysis and the use of skills. However, pressures to shift to more centralized forms of reporting continue.

information flows, intermediate management levels had to aggregate data from multiple facilities in the administrative unit to arrive at a report. With all its drudgery and imperfections, it still allowed for the managers to develop insights into the patterns of performance. Now as data flowed past them (directly into the national server), they not only lost these insights, but also data ownership, and refused to be held responsible for its reliability. The central systems responded by asking mid-level managers to sign in a confirmation of data, but to their surprise, there was a curious and obstinate reluctance, delay, and disobedience in doing so.

The second observation is that even within the logic of central monitoring, there is a need to understand the relationship of data elements to indicators and their underlying hierarchy. What we have in the existing design is a massive flow where every data element reaches the national level in the same form as it was at the point of collection. In theory, and in the administrator's perception, this is a good thing because by mapping trends in monthly measurements, they could understand facility performance. Such a perception is in some way intuitive for statisticians who rely on statistical outliers in trend measurements as the main basis of interpretation, and the ability to see the last mile is reassuring.

But reality is often counter-intuitive, and the administrators' intuitive understandings could be well off the mark. In practice there are no facility-wise denominators in the system to measure key indicators, limiting the derivation of meaning for a data element. Thus a facility report of providing 25 to 30 children with a measles vaccination in a month without mentioning a denominator, does not allow for interpreting whether the achievement is 50 per cent or 90 per cent, a very bad performance, or a very good one. There are instances when a district has shown a decline in immunization, when all they were doing was adjusting from an unrealistic 130 per cent immunization coverage to a more believable 100 per cent. Statistical outliers are not always data errors, but maybe a source of valuable information when one is measuring, say, drug stocks, when indicated stock-outs should stimulate action. Indeed, the large excess of non-usable data at the national levels provides a noise that clouds use of information, validating Finagle's law of the gap between wants and real needs.

Furthermore, though it seems common sense to assume that facility-based or name-based reporting would avoid the possibility of false reporting inherent when aggregate numbers are reported on, in practice, the increased granularity of information had no relevance to increasing data reliability, nor to its use for health programme management.

Clearly the lessons for designers would be to design systems to cater to the needs of the peripheral provider and the mid-level manager, and if this is well done, the information needs at top management and governance levels would become available as collateral. The needs of the service provider are essentially to document each service as and when it is provided, required for measuring the work s/he has done as well as resources (that s/he has consumed. drugs, consumables, etc.). The second need of the service provider is to have individual patient or client-specific records to enable building case history to support better quality of follow-up, indicating the quality of care provided. A third need is to be able to aggregate case-based data and provide reports upwards to help take resource allocation decisions, establish accountability, measure coverage, or undertake disease surveillance. Whether on paper or digitized, it is rare to find an example where all these needs are adequately taken care of.

The needs of the facility/hospital manager are similar. They need to document the work done, build up case histories to enable follow-up, and report to both management and public health authorities at the district. But in addition, there is also the organization and supervision of work processes and resource allocation within the facility. The larger and more complex the facility, the greater is this need, and in a large tertiary care hospital with over a 1000 beds, the needs of administration support to patient care may overwhelm all other needs. But despite this, the need for contributing to the population-based database does not reduce—on the contrary, it increases since large hospitals are handling a significant part of the healthcare burden of the region. The district manager needs to get more aggregated data than the facility managers in order to develop the overall picture of data quality coverage and health status of the catchment population. S/he is responsible for generating and transmitting feedback reports to the facilities, informing them of their achievement with respect to time, other facilities, and to the district and state, in addition to reporting district aggregate data to national level, to help assess programme performance, and to report to global agencies.

It follows that we need a system built around indicators to analyse facility or subdistrict performance, which are more useful than raw data elements. Reporting systems should put in place a hierarchy of indicators, at varying levels of granularity, to avoid equal emphasis on every indicator. To enable this, the IT systems in use—and the software/hardware configuration—requires functionalities to meet the information needs of the service provider and facility manager, as different from the district manager and policy maker. There is then the challenge of building capacity to analyse and use these indicators, which we discuss through another case.

Ten years back when computerized information systems were starting out, the differences between indicators and data elements were not properly understood. The limitations of working with data elements, as compared to its conversion into indicators, are now relatively well understood, although not equally well practised. Most public health programmes use a log-frame approach to monitoring which emphasizes the use of indicators. Most information systems therefore aim to build dashboards with limited indicators. There is a related set of problems regarding choosing or crafting the right indicators, and putting in place a hierarchy, so that most information flows up as indicators and only some as raw data elements. These are important issues, not discussed in this book, as these have been elaborated in various texts, and knowledge on this area has improved vastly in the last 10 years (Braa and Sahay 2012).

3.2 **Data Quality Issues: Beyond False Reporting**

A key learning from the Odisha case study relates to data quality. One set of issues relates to the structure and meaning of data itself. Data definitions can be taken for granted, whereas interpretations on the ground can be widely different. Thus, some facilities may include routine antenatal care and immunization services in the outpatient headcounts and others may leave them out, making measures of outpatient attendance meaningless. Or counting the day care admissions for a few hours along with other inpatients may make bed occupancy figures impossible to interpret. It is surprising how little of such variations in interpretation are recognized at both the provider and the managerial levels—since each is sure of their own version of the truth—and seldom listens to other versions. Confronted repeatedly with specific examples of divergence in definitions and the havoc they do to interpretation, managements concede the need for standardization, but then get surprised by the vigour with which different parties defend their version of the truth.

Today in many LMICs, national indicator sets with definitions are well established, such as in South Africa and Thailand. Data dictionaries have been developed as a document of standard reference. Recently, as part of the discussions on the post-2015 agenda, the World Health Organization (WHO 2015) has constituted a set of 100 global health indicators from which nations can choose according to their priorities within defined frameworks of standardization.

Another major contributor to poor data quality is the artefacts in use for primary recording of data. Most primary care providers use a set of registers that do not lend themselves to performing all three needs: recording, enabling patient follow-up—also referred to (unfortunately) as tracking, and aggregation for reporting. Usually efforts at register design prioritize one or the other— usually the tracking function—leaving the provider fumbling or even guessing, or innovating at random (e.g. drawing columns by hand in the register) to meet the other needs. At the hospital level, while the systems may be effective to record individual events, they are often woefully inadequate to develop aggregates from this individual data. Thus even apparently simple data, like the proportion of mothers who breastfed their newborns within the first hour, become almost impossible to obtain as the primary care register often does not provide a column to enter this. And at the hospital, the nurse's bed-head notes or doctor's case sheet would record it—but this is part of the details that do not flow to the hospital data manager. The final number reported is thus often an informed 'guesstimate'.

Population-based data is always constructed by aggregating data from multiple individual providers and facilities, or patient encounters. Ideally all facilities should not only report, but do so in a timely and complete manner. For indicators it is not only the numerators, but the denominators that also need to be aggregated. Technical solutions for the interoperability of aggregated information are surprisingly slow to develop, and there is more discussion on this than on practical working solutions. While software solutions are becoming smarter in providing validation rules for error checks, institutional protocols lag behind in fixing a process and the required human responsibility to act on the problems identified by the software, such as flagging violations of validation rules.

For those interested in data use, the simple message is this: do not wait for data to be perfect—start using the data—and in the process of using it, the quality of data would improve. However, for technical and institutional reasons, this vicious cycle is difficult to penetrate. This is now illustrated through a case study from a hospital information project in India (Case Study 3.2).

3.2.1 **Learnings from the Himachal case study**

Himachal Pradesh provides some very insightful learnings, useful for both rich, and low and middle-income countries. A key learning is the advantage of bottom-up and incremental approaches to hospital information systems development, as contrasted with large-scale, top-down efforts as exemplified by health information exchanges which we will also discuss in Chapter 4. The second is the use of a participatory approach, where the users take ownership of the system right from the design phase and where there are benefits to users at all levels. For the provider it is the support to care provision; for the administrator and public health specialist it is population-based data. The third learning concerns the length of time required to implement such complex systems. The state gave HISP India more than five years for the project, which allowed the system to mature, and the state gradually took ownership of the system. The system still continues, and the state has been visionary in providing the system this time and space to do so.

Another important learning from both the Himachal and the Odisha case studies is the importance of establishing conversations over data between different key players—the programme managers, administrators, providers, and the health management information systems (HMIS) managers. This helps us

(continued on page 63)

Case Study 3.2 Hospital Information System, Himachal Pradesh, India

A hospital information system including an EMR (electronic medical record) is what many LMICs are currently trying to introduce in their historically neglected public hospitals. The patient record theoretically captures details of an individual patient over time, and is capable of being shared within and across facilities. There are different models of sharing and architecture possible, from standalone servers in facilities which can be synced in batch mode to a central server, or through centralized databases. Examples of the latter is what many countries, rich and poor, are striving to achieve, but with very poor results and at a high cost. Patient data could include demographics, medical history, medication and allergies, immunization status, laboratory test results, radiology images, vital signs, personal statistics like age and weight, and billing information. The unsolved challenge of this individual data is how to aggregate it to develop population-based statistics.

In 2010, the government of Himachal Pradesh, a northern mountainous state in India, decided to develop an integrated hospital information system including EMRs, and to deploy it across their 20 district and subdistrict hospitals to strengthen clinical care, improve hospital management and administration, and ensure continuity of care to patients. This was also important to shift some of the patient load from hospitals to primary care levels.

Developing population-based aggregates was not part of the original agenda. After an initial scoping and negotiation exercise, 10 priority modules were identified, including registration, billing, outpatient and inpatient departments (OPD and IPD), pharmacy, stocks, laboratory, blood bank, and reports. A reference hospital was chosen where these modules would be implemented on an incremental basis, and which would become the standard for the remaining 19 hospitals. In addition, an integration module based on global standards was also proposed, to aggregate patient-level data, and to export that into the existing data warehouse in use as the state HMIS application, DHIS 2, in order to develop state-level aggregate reports for various health programmes.

The project was initiated in September 2010, when the government contracted an Indian NGO, HISP India, to carry out the entire project where capacity building of all hospital staff across the 20 facilities was an integral part.

The project adopted an open source platform called OpenMRS, and used a participatory approach to design. In the first year, HISP India developed these 10 modules and implemented them in the reference hospital with strong accompanying processes of capacity building and hand-holding support. Indeed, much of the investment went into the capacity building. After installation and six months of intensive support, the system started to be used regularly, although not all the modules. The application was then replicated to six other hospitals by the end of the second year. There were delays due to problems of hardware procurement, and the establishment of the local area network in the hospitals, as there are some cumbersome processes for government procurement, but eventually these were managed.

In September 2013, the state decided to take over from the hospitals the responsibility for the procurement and networking. In this phase, HISP India was given a one-year period to roll out the application in 11 further facilities, which they did, except for three hospitals that got cut off in winter due to snow. These three hospitals were later covered by the end of 2014. Despite this full state coverage, both the state and HISP India were concerned with the limited use of the application, especially the modules for outpatient and inpatient care. A survey was undertaken to assess the reasons for this suboptimal use. Seven hospitals were surveyed, and the survey team had interactions with system users, administrators, and patients. The key learning was that only the registration and billing modules were running effectively across all the hospitals, primarily because their work process was integrated well with the computerization. The registration process required data entry and there was a person available to do this; similarly with generation of the bills. These personnel had no external tasks. Hardware and networking did pose problems. For example, non-functional printers, stolen hard disks and keyboards, and frequent change of rooms requiring new networking caused difficulties and severely impeded use of some modules. Registration and billing were relatively spared these problems, as someone was responsible for their use.

The problems with IT support for clinical and ancillary services were more acute. Here entering data into the system, and using the information for clinical decision-making had to be done by the same providers, and manpower issues were a challenge. The nurses and lab technicians were overburdened with everyday work, and did not find the time or the incentive to use the system. Furthermore, the state had issued no formal directive to make the system mandatory, thus allowing for the manual and hospital information system to run in parallel, making data entry an additional work burden. In addition, laboratory technicians already had lab analysers working, which provided electronic results as a print out. Since the new system was not integrated to it, the technicians were reluctant to enter the same data thrice (in manual records, in the analysers, and in the hospital information system). The biggest resistance to use came from the doctors, whose reluctance to use the OPD and IPD modules adversely affected the running of the overall system.

The doctors attributed this reluctance to their high workloads (going up to 100 patients a day, giving a doctor two to three minutes to see a patient), and their poor computer skills for the rapid entry that was required. Use somewhat improved when doctors were given options to enter the full patient record or a part, or just the diagnosis, and they could choose to enter data for those patients where longitudinal follow-up was needed. One also has to reckon with a deeper problem. In routine practice, often treatment is presumptive and based on suspected diagnosis. Sometimes there are multiple diagnoses suspected and a broad spectrum treatment covers all. There is considerable uncertainty regarding diagnosis and response to treatment. Under such circumstances, doctors often try different treatments until something works. Furthermore, in the crowded outpatient departments a sort of triage occurs, wherein only patients with a certain degree of sickness attract a full medical check-up. Others are managed symptomatically. In such a context, entry of all details into the patient record, with an International Classification of Diseases (ICD) coded diagnosis, gives the uncertainty a certain solidity and definitiveness that the doctor is not ready for. With computerization, the paperwork largely remains, and patient care does not become easier, only adding one more layer of work. Governance of the system from both the state and the hospital was weak, with limited ownership, no control over transfer of trained manpower, and absence of clear directives from the state to the hospital on what kind of use was expected from them.

In the third phase, HISP India took up conducting refresher trainings in all hospitals to try and strengthen ownership and stimulate processes of use. Prior to the trainings, baseline assessments were undertaken for each hospital to understand the existing situation, and to help design solutions. First hardware and network issues were addressed by verifying LAN points and the functioning of other hardware, which included such details as physically switching on and off every computer, checking power points, printers, the availability of printing paper, the functioning of browsers on each computer, and so on. Hospital staff were given the phone numbers of facilitators and were encouraged to call and when they needed help, and not to wait for a senior to intervene or for any administrative process to complete.

Once this was done, based on the gaps identified, focused capacity building was carried out. Data were presented to the hospitals on systems usage in their hospital, as well as comparisons on the same indicators with other facilities. This was expected to stimulate interest in interpreting the information and motivation for action.

Simultaneous to the efforts at the hospital level, the HISP India senior management started to meet with the state administrators to argue for data-use workshops, whereby hospital and state administrators could be shown their information. Initially, the state were reluctant, arguing that there was not enough good quality data in the system to have a meaningful workshop. But the team pointed out the relationship between quality and use, and that taking by data seriously was to enhance its use. This workshop also became useful for the state to reiterate directives to the hospitals that use of the system is mandatory, and they would be provided all the support they needed to materialize meaningful use.

Various issues were highlighted by the doctors, one being around registration. It was pointed out that owing to long queues, the data entry operator never asks whether the patient is new or existing, and would register most as new unless the patient had documentary proof of the previous visit. For reasons of expediency, registration clerks were avoiding details like phone number, name of relative, and area of domicile, which could have helped as identifiers. This absence of details led to duplication of records and defied the key benefit of a longitudinal medical record of a patient. So, while ideally in a hospital revisits are estimated at 20 to 30 per cent of the total, it was found that the actual figures were less than 10 per cent.

Similarly, inpatient data had its own set of issues. Data on deliveries did not report on complications and relevant in-hospital health events, although this was written on bed-head notes. This lack of reporting did not allow determining the number of Caesarean sections, and other complications requiring varied management responses. This lack of data was attributed to the workload of the ward sisters who were to do the data entry, and their limited computer literacy. The data also showed many cases of cataract surgeries, but the count of surgeries did not include them. However, when the data were used as a performance measure during a discussion, the doctors protested the under-reporting, but were motivated to be more careful in the data entry in the future which would add value to their information.

After the workshop, OPD attendance figures showed a rise. The data-use workshop was held in May, and the figures in June suggested some improvements in usage. While attendance by OPD figures was always available with manual records, this was aggregated by patient encounters, and could now be technically combined with other electronic data to add new value. Zuboff (1987) indentifes this as the difference between automate and informate. Information about proportional caseloads can be correlated with information on workforce deployment or consumption of consumables for the potentially better allocation of resources. Further 'informate' value can be created by transferring data from the hospital information system to the state DHIS 2 data warehouse to generate population-based indicators. How this was achieved is discussed in Chapter 4 on integration.

to understand and improve data quality, and interpret and use information for action. A vicious negative cycle now gets converted into a positive feedback of improvement. It generates a different culture about information and knowledge itself, one embedded in a more realist philosophical tradition, where meanings are made of information only in context, which inform action, and where there is constant learning from this process. Finally it emphasizes again that information generation, analytics, and use is a multifaceted problem comprising issues of infrastructure, technology, governance, individual behaviour, workloads, capacity, and many others. In short, it is a health systems challenge, and needs to be addressed in the same framework; otherwise, results will always be suboptimal.

We now turn to the issue of capacity strengthening to enable information use. We start with a case study from Zanzibar, Tanzania, and then discuss some learning from it with reference to capacity (Case Study 3.3).

3.2.2 **Learnings from the Zanzibar case study**

The outcomes of the data-use workshops validate the hypothesis that the more data are used, the more data quality will improve, leading to significant innovations in the use of information and breaking the vicious cycle of non-use and poor quality of data.

This case study also explains what a more holistic understanding of organizational capacity implies. It is the acquisition of necessary skills, certainly. But it is also the establishment of certain formal and informal rules of how things are done (data-use workshops, self-assessment, peer-critique, readiness to converse over data etc.) and an enabling environment for these practices to flourish. Zanzibar health systems can therefore be said to have developed the capacity to use information. While we find similar features in the Odisha

(continued on page 66)

Case Study 3.3 The Case of Zanzibar: Capacity Strengthening As a Key Enabler of Information Use

Zanzibar, in the United Republic of Tanzania, provides an example of how peer reviewed data-use workshops can be an approach to address problems of data quality and data use simultaneously. This case study further reinforces the hypothesis that data quality and data use are interrelated: poor quality data will not be used, and because they are not used, the data will remain of poor quality; conversely, greater use of data will help to improve their quality, which will in turn lead to more data use. This hypothesis was tested through data-use workshops involving systematic peer review, building teamwork, and stimulating self-assessment, and using indicators to measure targets.

Zanzibar consists of two islands, each making up a health zone; one island comprises six districts and the other four. As part of a health system strengthening project, in 2005 the HMIS Unit of the Ministry of Health, with support from the Danish International Development Agency, launched a process aimed at strengthening the HMIS, improving data reporting, and implementing the DHIS v1.

Quarterly data-use workshops were held, in which district health management team (DHMT) members (roughly seven per district) presented their district's routine data to their peers from other districts. The workshops lasted approximately five days each and were facilitated by external facilitators from the Health Information Systems Programme, supported by the Zanzibar HMIS Unit and selected health zone staff. The workshops began in 2005 and have continued since then. Most workshops are now being run by the HMIS Unit without outside help. During the workshops, each district or programme presented and assessed its own data using standardized analysis templates based on the Millennium Development Goals (MDGs) and local strategic plans, after which their peers discussed and critiqued these presentations in order to encourage self-assessment, provide opportunities to compare presentations, identify common issues relating to data quality and health services performance, promote local involvement, and improve data quality. They also contributed with direct feedback to HMIS planners for the revision of indicators and data sets and to software developers for the design of new functionalities, reports, and other features.

These workshops contributed to the simplification of forms based on revised indicators, dramatically reducing the number of data elements collected and thus the workload of facility staff. This simplification was achieved largely because workshop participants realized that it was unnecessary to disaggregate some data (e.g. by age, sex, or uncommon diseases) which were not being used. Similarly, duplication of data collection by different programmes was virtually eliminated (e.g. the Reproductive and Child Health Programme stopped collecting data on HIV infection, immunization, and malaria) and data gaps were filled. Changes were agreed collectively through improved communication fostered by the workshops and supported by strong leadership from the Ministry of Health.

Data submission improved considerably, with districts reporting more regularly on most data forms. The process began modestly, focusing on a couple of programmes, but other programmes gradually saw the value of using the national HMIS rather than their own parallel data collection systems, and more programmes (and hospitals, including the national referral hospital) were added. Indicator set changes, including some reductions in indicators, were negotiated with programmes jointly each year through the HMIS Unit, HISP, and the two health zones.

The workshops provided a stimulus for integration of the previously separate data sets and databases of PHC units, hospitals and programmes, and allowed the DHMTs to gain a better idea of the roles played by different actors, which improved practical collaboration. Integration of programme data into a single DHIS database—with one national data set covering the MDG indicators, poverty reduction, and national strategic plan indicators, and programme-specific indicators—was a major achievement. Integration was a slow process, however, as some externally funded programmes were initially reluctant to share 'their' data and did not trust the quality, or timeliness of the national database.

Data quality improved dramatically, thanks to increased use of quality checks (for timeliness, correctness, consistency, and completeness of data) at the facility level, use of computer checks by districts and practical experience gained under supervision during workshops. Mistakes were identified by participants when data were presented during workshops, sometimes leading to heated discussion of quality issues, which made a strong impression on participants. At the start of the process, most DHMT staff did not think in terms of indicators, and their presentations focused on raw data. As these people became more competent in using the HMIS, data analysis tools (targets and indicators) became more widely used and understood, which strengthened self-assessment and 'epidemiological thinking'. The link between plans, targets, and indicators was emphasized, which helped to increase the use of indicators at local levels and the analysis of coverage and quality of service delivery. DHMT team members honed their ability to solve problems using HMIS data as they gained appreciation of the value of improved data quality, and felt more competent in applying epidemiological approaches to daily data management issues.

Teamwork improved considerably as the DHMT staff shared information about service delivery and used the HMIS to monitor and evaluate progress towards targets set in their district annual plans. Leaders became more confident in making evidence-based decisions to improve quality of care based on collective values developed through the data-use workshops. While a 'culture of information' takes time to establish, clearly significant strides were made in that direction. Workshop participants improved their computer skills in using DHIS for analysis, presentation, and dissemination, and also enhanced their knowledge of basic hardware and software maintenance. DHMT members' presentation skills were initially weak, as they were unused to drawing graphs, using PowerPoint, engaging in debate, or offering constructive criticism. These skills improved dramatically as a result of the workshops, especially when standardized templates for presentations were developed. Local HMIS Unit and health zone personnel acquired sufficient skills to run the workshops without outside facilitators.

Adapted from Braa J, Heywood A, and Sahay S. Improving quality and use of data through data-use workshops: Zanzibar, United Republic of Tanzania. *Bulletin of the World Health Organization*, Volume 90, pp. 379-384, Copyright © 2012 WHO.

and Himachal case studies too, they were not as fully developed and stabilized as in Zanzibar. The main difference is that in the Indian case studies, these actions were often done as special one-time correctives, whereas in Zanzibar it is established as the necessary and institutional way of how data is to be used. The peer review-based approach helped to establish 'a community of practice'. When critique is only external or by supervisory staff, similar progress is not made, and practices cannot be institutionalized.

The better use of information in Zanzibar leads not only to benefits in strengthening health systems and outcomes, but also to improvements in the information systems themselves—in terms of better data collection, rationalization of information flows, and a breakdown of the barriers which had impeded the integration of parallel information systems. Clearly better use of information can drive changes for improved information systems, turning the usual intuitive understanding on its head.

3.3 **The Politics of Information Use: Beyond Traditional Rationalities**

There are other barriers to better use of information. It is now commonly recognized that use of information exclusively for monitoring—to find gaps to which the management must respond by suitable disciplinary action—is counterproductive to reliability of information and to its use. If all a primary care provider can get in return for the extra effort involved in reporting regularly is reprimand for any failings, the message s/he gets is to hide the bad news, which makes the whole purpose of the exercise fruitless.

But could this logic also be operating at the systemic level—in macropolicy? If we postulate that the government makes very good policies, which are poorly implemented, and such poor implementation is by errant peripheral providers, then we arrive at one type of systems design—one that is guided by control logic. In a control logic, the HMIS is a tool of constant surveillance of the workforce—a panopticon, in the sense that Micheal Foucault uses the term (Foucault 1975). It sets out a grid of expected actions, behaviours, and reports from the workforce. It is not the actual analysis and use that leads to change, but the very existence of such an all-seeing eye would bring about the desired behaviour change. In one extension of this monitoring logic, an innovation in the use of information and communications technologies for monitoring actually built in a CCTV camera into every subcentre, so that the service providers felt they were constantly under the supervisory gaze. Needless to say, it made no difference; and as common with all panopticons, the central watchtower is either empty, or does not have the capacity to see and take action.

But, if on the other hand, the failings on the ground are really reflective of management or governance failures, then the HMIS design is only a way of shifting accountability. A functional HMIS which is correctly interpreted would point fingers upwards at the leadership and its failures. The information visible may not be consistent with the face that those in power would like to present to the public. Such information would make the leadership very uncomfortable and set limits to the desire to use information.

A recent example was a series of exposes in *The Economist* (2015), which leaked and published the entire data set regarding a rapid survey of children carried out by UNICEF in India. What was curious is that actually the data showed remarkable improvement in malnutrition and immunization parameters. *The Economist* attributed this reluctance of the Indian government to celebrate its success to the fact that a cross-state analysis did not support the currently dominant political view of which economic policies are better in terms of equity and human development. On the contrary, it seemed to be implicitly supporting policies of the earlier government.

It is always difficult to establish whether this is indeed the cause of reluctance to share data. A reluctance or discomfort with the truth at the intermediate leadership levels could explain the under-reporting of maternal and child deaths by routine HMIS across all LMICs, and in reporting of vaccine preventable disease outbreaks and deaths. Or increases in deaths or disease prevalence could be corelated with lack of key supplies or failure to recruit staff, or make the necessary investments.

In most LMICs, government investments on health sector are suboptimal, and its policies too narrowly focused on a few priorities which international aid agencies and local elite have a disproportionate voice in determining. A large number of the deaths and diseases that take place in these nations are preventable and one could postulate that any meaningful use of information would only make this more apparent and actionable. It is *not* our contention that there is a conspiracy to suboptimally develop and use information systems. In that respect, we would differ from the implications of *The Economist*'s articles. But a good institutional analysis could provide insights on the links between co-relations of power and choices made with regard to what purposes of information systems dominate and which uses of information are marginalized, which areas of knowledge are gathered and receive focus, and which are ignored—and why there is a divergence between the almost obsessive-compulsive collection of information and the stagnation and relative neglect in its use.

3.4 The Way Forward: How the Expanded PHI Approach Engages with the Use of Information Problematic

The existing solutions to this problem of strengthening use have come through initiatives of improving data quality, streamlining and standardizing data sets, and building better dashboards for visualization and analysis. While these are important steps and need to be further strengthened, they remain incomplete as they represent largely technical solutions. The Expanded PHI approach guides us to a broader and more systemic view within a health systems framework. We do this in three ways. One is through a focus on *conversations around data*, which seeks to create broader structures for change. The second is through *communities of practice*, which seeks to provide enabling forums in which these conversations should take place. The third is the need to integrate IT solutions more effectively into the work processes of the care provider. These approaches are elaborated upon next.

Conversations around data represent people, practices, and tools used to work with data, and in our case the focus is on work around the analysis, use, and dissemination of data. Currently these conversations take place typically at the central levels, involving primarily statisticians, working with statistical tools and approaches, largely within a top-down culture to show up problems in data quality, and to create annual statistical yearbooks. Within such a framework, it is impossible to bring about conversations that will promote meaningful information use. In trying to redefine these frameworks, four issues become important. *Who* participates, *where* these conversations take place, *what* is the content of these conversations, and *how* they are enabled.

With respect to the question of *who*, it is important to broaden participation by including programme's workers (currently the data, IT, and statistics people dominate), and also the broader civil society. Only through this broadening can we include the voices of those responsible for providing care and its beneficiaries. Such a focus can shift the historically existing vertical channels of conversation, to also incorporate horizontal flows, for example across different health programmes in the district. The *where* of these conversations needs to shift from the centre to the periphery where care is transacted and can thus be meaningfully debated, and to public places (like media, newspapers, public forums, and information portals) for highlighting that health is an issue of the public, not just the state, and that the voices of the population should shape healthcare processes. The *what* question is intimately linked to the content of the conversation and concerns questions of accountability and transparency. The state tends to 'black-box' issues of public health relevance, revealing little, and often; and, as the case of the nutrition survey in India suggests, information may be deliberately withheld from public consumption. Not only does such information of relevance need to be made accessible to civil society, it needs to be debated, and implications for public health carefully articulated. The *how* question is important to consider, as it may lead to inclusion or exclusion of certain groups of people from the conversations. For example, illiterate populations without access to computing resources, whose health is of fundamental importance in the public health context, may tend to be excluded from online conversations about their own conditions. More context-sensitive and appropriate mechanisms to enable their participation need to be considered.

A focus on conversations around data, we argue, will help to shift the focus from the positivist view of 'evidence-based' decision-making, to the shaping of realist discourses which can promote a broader information culture, where the terms in which the production, distribution, and consumption of information contribute to how information is valued and what changes it brings about. The focus would then be on practices of how and what information is collected, used, and disseminated, rather than some search for an elusive absolute and singular version of the truth, which has as its corollaries the issue of power and authority to decide on the access and interpretation of such information. A recognition that there are many, often contradictory, interests at work, and all data and its interpretation has political implications beyond its use for the good of public health, should encourage us to institutionalize 'conversations over data' at every level as the way to improve both use and quality of data. And there is an urgent need to broaden the participation in these conversations, so as to lift the quality of the conversations to enable meaningful information use, rather than leaving it at the mercy of the technical specialists and politicians. These conversations are not one-time remedial measures to achieve data fidelity, but are part of the routine and systemic way in which use of information is institutionalized, becoming part of a learning and adaptive system which is forever improving itself.

Our second broad approach is a corollary of the first and calls for building communities of practice as a vehicle and forum, for not only enabling meaningful conversations, but for building information systems as well. Communities of practice represent people who are engaged in achieving similar goals, and in our case, enabling more effective use of information. These communities can be comprised of health programme managers, district teams (as the Zanzibar case illustrates), academics and researchers, systems designers, IT developers, information scientists, civil society groups, and private providers. A simple principle guiding the value of such communities is that we learn better in collectives than in isolated singular settings, and by sharing best practices, resources, experiences, and innovations within the community, we can avoid reinventing the wheel, and thus shorten the learning curve. Many such collectives are now visible, such as open source software development communities, which share ideas on software design and development. Creating specific interest groups around information use can greatly provide impetus to our efforts, and expand participation in these debates.

The final principle of design that we consider as non-negotiable is establishing use of information at the level of healthcare providers, who are also the data collectors. Unless the collection of data is integrated into their work processes and brings value to their work, in the form of either reducing drudgery and effort of recording and reporting on data, or enabling them to improve the quality of care they provide, or in providing new insights into their process and outcomes—reliable data would be difficult to come by.

These principles of IT's integration into the work processes of the care provider, conversations around data, and communities of practice thus become three important design principles in the Expanded PHI approach that we are arguing for in this book.

3.5 **References**

Braa, J., and Sahay, S. (2012). *Integrated Health Information Architecture: Power for the Users: Design Development and Use*. Matrix Publishing, New Delhi, India.

Chambers, R. (1983). *Rural Development: Putting the Last First*. Longman, London, UK.

Foucault, M. (1975). *Discipline and Punish: The Birth of a Prison*. Random House, New York, NY.

Lippeveld, T., Sauerborn, R., and Bodart, C. (2000). *Design and Implementation of Health Information Systems*. World Health Organization, Geneva, Switzerland.

Sahay, S., and Walsham, G. (1996). Implementation of GIS in India: Organizational issues and implications. *International Journal of Geographical Information Systems*, **10**(4), 385–404.

Sahay, S. (1997). Implementation of information technology: a time-space perspective. *Organization Studies*, **18**(2), 229–60.

Suchman, L.A. (1987). *Plans and Situated Actions: The Problem of Human-Machine Communication*. Cambridge University Press, New York, NY.

The Economist (2015). Nutrition in India: Of secrecy and stunting. [Online]. Available at: http://www.economist.com/news/asia/21656709-government-withholds-report-nutrition-contains-valuable-lessons-secrecy-and [Last accessed: 1 October 2015].

WHO (2015). Towards a monitoring framework with targets and indicators for the health goals of the post-2015 Sustainable Development Goals. Draft discussion paper. [Online]. Available at: http://www.who.int/healthinfo/indicators/hsi_indicators_sdg_targetindicators_draft.pdf [Last accessed: 1 October 2015].

Zuboff, S. (1987). *In the Age of the Smart Machine*. Basic Books, New York, NY.

Chapter 4

The Challenge of Integration: (In)adequacy of Technical Solutions to Institutional Challenges

4.1 Integration in Public Health Informatics

In this chapter, we explore the wicked problem of fragmentation, and popular approaches to finding integration solutions to them. Most such solutions are driven primarily by technically focused logics. We explore the deeper reasons why such problems keep recurring, and why the currently available solutions remain insufficient. In the first section, we set up the fragmentation–integration problematic, arguing for more nuanced approaches for analysis and development of solutions. Next we explore the question of 'why' to understand the multiple logics that drive integration efforts. Following this, we analyse the question of 'how', referring to some contemporary approaches to address fragmentation, focusing on the Open Health Information Exchange, which is being presented as a modern solution to the integration problem in both rich nations and in low and middle-income countries (LMICs). Finally, we explore how the Expanded PHI approach can provide some novel insights to the problematic posed in this chapter.

4.2 The Problematic of Integration

Fragmentation is universally acknowledged as a fundamental problem plaguing LMICs' health information systems (HIS) in the contemporary context of ongoing health reforms (HMN 2008). Fragmentation is undoubtedly a 'wicked' problem, since trying to address it in one place may throw up new and unexpected issues in other places. Integration is positioned as a modern solution to this problem, and significant efforts and money are being put in by ministries, donors, software vendors, and others to try and address it.

This problem and the top-down approaches used to solve it are not unique to LMICs, but are also widespread in rich countries like the United States and the United Kingdom. A quick look at the landscape of these efforts highlights many stories of why integration did not work, interspersed with very few accounts of successful efforts, where significant organizational benefits can be said to have accrued. And yet the information community continues with these efforts, coming up with newer technologies and methodologies to address the same problems, with largely similar outcomes. Given the significance of the fragmentation problem, and the high attention and investment going into these efforts and the not-so-optimal outcomes, it is important to unpack the nature of this problematic, understand why this is the case, and explore how the Expanded PHI perspective can potentially provide a useful lens to explore alternative and more effective ways to approach this wicked problem.

Fragmentation from a computer science perspective concerns computer storage space being used inefficiently or being 'wasted', with adverse implications on capacity or performance—most often both. In sociology, fragmentation takes on a very different meaning. The context is about people and their social relations. Here fragmentation can refer to the absence or underdevelopment of linkages between different social groups and organizations. Such fragmentation can be due to culture, nationality, race, language, occupation, and income levels, or it could be due to the common interests and rules that bind them into an organization. Addressing such conditions of fragmentation is not a trivial challenge, as they are embedded in history, institutional legacies, and often invisible power structures and social norms and culture.

An Expanded PHI perspective informs us that the fragmentation problem is technical (as illustrated by the computer science perspective, or the focus on the individual patient devoid of social context), social (as seen from the sociology perspective), and also organizational (as seen from a managerial or governance perspective). These are usually intimately inter-connected and result in the poor performance of the entire system, a point often missed in designing integration solutions. In addition, fragmentation could occur due to the structure of disease control programmes, and the behaviour of different stakeholders like donors, or different departments and administrative levels within the government.

To illustrate these linkages (or the lack of them), we draw upon an example from a national initiative in India to implement the Mother and Child Tracking System (MCTS). This system aimed at tracking every pregnant mother, by name, and recording all the events of her maternity care lifecycle including details of each antenatal visits, events at delivery, and during postnatal care. The same system was also tasked to track every child by name over their immunization lifecycle, from the first vaccine to full immunization. This system was introduced in late 2009 in parallel to an existing health management information system (HMIS; as also described in the Odisha case study; see Case Study 3.1). The HMIS was collecting aggregate figures relating to pregnancy and immunization for a particular facility and time period. A driving logic for MCTS was one of accountability—in effect better command and control—as the health department stated that the aggregate numbers on the HMIS reported by the field staff were not trustworthy, and would improve if services were reported by individual names which were easier to cross-verify than aggregates. An elaborate system of a centralized national call centre in Delhi, from which verification calls would go out to a sample of the over 60 million pregnant women recorded on the tracking system, was part of the design.

The MCTS ran in parallel to the HMIS, with no inter-connections. Thus, the HMIS data continued to flow as aggregate numbers with no inputs from the MCTS, though in the stated logic one would have expected HMIS figures to allow only aggregate figures of MCTS. Many socio-technical dimensions of fragmentation are evident from this example, some more visible than others.

- Firstly, a *data-related* fragmentation, as a health worker had to report data of the same phenomenon (e.g. antenatal care) to two different information systems, one aggregate and the other name-based. The integration solution here could have been a relatively simple technical redesigning of the name-based data being aggregated, and then posting it into the HMIS as numbers. Further, this simple solution would require integration of computers (using the same machine for data entry), servers (using one source for data storage), and also of other supporting infrastructure like the internet.

- Secondly, there is a *technology-related* fragmentation, as the data on the MCTS could not be aggregated and transferred to the HMIS system. There were both semantic differences and technical problems that potentially could have been resolved, but to this day have not been.

- Thirdly, there was an organizational or *work-related* fragmentation. Due to the increasing data burden, care delivery activities got marginalized by the ever-increasing data work. The field nurse was to enter all the data onto a large specialized paper register for the MCTS, which was in addition to every register she was already maintaining. This register would then be transported, usually by the nurse herself, to the block or district headquarters, where a data entry operator would enter the data into the computer. More often than not, the nurse had to be present when this was being done. This required a relatively more complex integration solution of work rationalization, such as reallocating data-related work to someone other than the field nurse providing care, and withdrawing some of the other registers she had to maintain to reduce duplication.

- Fourthly, there is an *institution-related* fragmentation, as the logic of (health worker) control pulls the nurse further away from the institutional mandate of providing care for all on a larger package of services. Her work gets limited to what is in the MCTS register. This is a much more complex governance problem to address that is embedded in history (of bureaucratic control), hierarchy, technological imperatives, and donor interests (which promote the collection of individual-level data).

These different facets of the solution are necessarily inter-connected; for example, addressing work-related fragmentation solutions must necessarily consider solutions of data-level integration, and seek institutional corrections which downplay control-based logics. The problematic is thus multilayered (going from the global to the individual), multifaceted, and dynamically unfolding over time.

All compartmentalization of data flows need not be a 'fragmentation' and negative in impact. For example, the logic of a disease and its control programme may call for stand-alone rather than integrated efforts. Disease epidemics do not know district-level boundaries, and often require central national-driven efforts, rather than a district system where the necessary specialization and expertise to deal with the disease may be limited. Questioning the why of integration, and the inherent (often irreconcilable) complexities that may be involved, urges the need for more cautious approaches to integration, rather than shooting off the hip with largely technical 'one size fits all' solutions. Stand-alone systems should often be accepted in return for simplicity or avoiding triggering of something worse than the status quo. But even then one would need means to talk to them. After all, this is a wicked problem!

4.3 **The Why (or not) of Integration**

The 'why' for integration comes from multiple governance-related sources, including international declarations, national strategies, and empirical experiences where senior managers realize the inadequacy of the data at hand in relation to their information needs, primarily due to fragmentation of data sources, inefficient information flows, poor computer systems, high work burden arising from duplication of data collection, and poor analysis, as all required data is not available in one place. Realization of this fragmentation problem leads to a variety of integration efforts ranging from rationalization of data sources to remove redundancies, making uniform data flows, sharing data between systems, creating shared data resources, and developing unified governance frameworks.

In the mid-1990s, as a part of the post-apartheid South African health sector reconstruction and development process, the government in South Africa worked towards the design of a district-based data warehouse to enable decentralization. In that extreme of racial, organizational, and social fragmentation, authorities quickly realized that the existing data flows from various facility-based sources, each going to their racially and programmatically fragmented authorities outside the district, needed to be consolidated in one central point within the district, where it could be accessed and used by the newly formed district health management teams. Such a functional model for integration was subsequently pursued by various international agencies such as the Health Metrics Network (HMN) through their data warehouse framework, which many countries adopted into their HIS planning processes, but largely failed to subsequently implement.

There have been various conventions and international commitments emphasizing integration that LMICs have signed up to, such as the World Summit on Information Society and resolutions in the 58th and 66th World Health Assembly. Furthermore, many countries (Rwanda, Philippines, Bangladesh, India, and others) have in national policy statements defined integration to be a cornerstone of their national HIS efforts. Some examples are provided of such international imperatives which emphasize integration:

- The World Summit on Information Society declaration (2003) said, among other things:
  - Alert, monitor, and control the spread of communicable diseases, through the improvement of common information systems.
  - Promote the development of international standards for the exchange of health data, taking due account of privacy issues and concerns.
- The 58th World Health Assembly (WHO 2005), urged member states to:
  - Draw up a long-term strategic plan for developing and implementing e-health services in various areas of health sectors including health administration, which includes an appropriate legal framework and infrastructure and encourages public and private partnership.
  - Mobilize multisectoral collaboration for determining evidence-based e-health standards and norms and to share the knowledge of cost-effective models, thus ensuring quality, safety, and ethical standards, and respect for the principles of confidentiality of information, privacy, equity, and equality.
  - Establish national centres and networks of excellence for e-health best practice, policy coordination, and technical support for healthcare

delivery, service improvement, information to citizens, capacity building, and surveillance.

◆ On the same lines, the 66th World Health Assembly (WHO 2013) urged member states to:

  • Consider options to collaborate with relevant stakeholders, including national authorities, relevant ministries, healthcare providers, and academic institutions, in order to draw up a road map for implementation of e-health and health data standards at national and subnational levels.
  • To ensure compliance in adoption of e-health and health data standards by public and private sectors, as appropriate, and the donor community, as well as to ensure the privacy of personal clinical data.

Currently, the world is moving towards defining shared health goals for post-2015 development agenda. Various agencies are jointly involved in these integration efforts to create this shared agenda. The World Health Organization, the World Bank, and the United States Agency for International Development (USAID), with support from the Bill & Melinda Gates Foundation, are seeking to construct a common strategy to improve and sustain country accountability systems for health results in the post-2015 era. This strategy aims to: (a) take stock of the current state of the systems for measurement and accountability for health results; (b) to identify innovative approaches and strategic investments that can strengthen health data availability, quality, and use; and (c) agree on a common roadmap for health measurement and accountability in the context of the post-2015 agenda (the World Bank 2015). In June 2015, these organizations jointly convened a global summit at the World Bank headquarters in the United States, to discuss with governments, multilateral agencies, and civil society to produce a roadmap for health measurement and accountability, and identify investments that countries can adopt to strengthen basic measurement systems.

These international calls have emphasized the need for stronger integration through intra- and multisectoral coordination, building and adhering to standards, and building unified systems for data collection, reporting, and measuring accountability. There is thus a global acknowledgement that integration is much more than a technical problem.

Moving from these globally driven agendas and logics shaping integration, we discuss some empirical examples from countries to illustrate the more national and field-driven logics.

4.3.1 National integration efforts in India

A large-scale national-level HMIS reform effort was undertaken by the Indian Ministry of Health starting in 2008, and here we present some snippets of this extensive and long-term effort to illustrate some of the reasons underlying integration efforts. This HMIS integration was embedded within a broader health systems reform agenda initiated within the framework of the National Rural Health Mission (NRHM) which sought to strengthen the country's public health systems. By design, NRHM aimed at architectural corrections in the health systems through integration, decentralization, and strengthening evidence-based decision-making. HMIS integration was intimately interlinked with this broader reform agenda.

An initial process of redesign of the recording and reporting formats ensued, where the effort was to develop single reporting formats for different facility types (subcentre, primary health centre, and district hospitals), as compared to the then existing different programme-based data reporting forms at each facility type. Without discussing the entire redesign process, four examples from India are described which illustrate the interplay of different logics. The first two examples are from the national level, while the third, presented as Case Study 4.1, is from the state of Tamil Nadu, and Case Study 4.2 is from Himachal Pradesh.

The first example concerned the integration of the IDSP (Integrated Disease Surveillance Programme), which reports on notifiable diseases on a weekly basis, with a routine HMIS which reports on facility-based services and health status conditions on a monthly basis. There were a number of meetings held at the national level between the monitoring and evaluation (M&E) division representing the HMIS and the IDSP programme managers, and the World Health Organization (WHO) that was supporting them. These meetings were chaired by a senior bureaucrat (the Mission Director) who was heading up the NRHM. In these discussions, the IDSP rejected the idea of integration, using the argument that IDSP data inscribed a 'surveillance logic', which was different as compared to HMIS because, firstly, it carried a weekly frequency (as compared to monthly frequency for HMIS), and secondly, 'zero' reports of data values had significant meaning since it implied an absence of disease as compared to HMIS, where a zero could mean that the field has been left blank. The HMIS argument that this logic could be incorporated in the existing system and integration would lead to improved coverage of IDSP reporting was not accepted, leading to a failure of the integration effort in the design phase itself. This failure to integrate could be seen to reflect conflicting logics of the *health programme* of IDSP and that of the HMIS *statistical data*.

Our second example, from the same national-level Indian effort, was of integrating the EPI (Expanded Programme on Immunization) with the HMIS, which had significant duplications in immunization data collection.

For example, measles data was being collected in three places: HMIS, IDSP, and EPI (which used software called RIMS—Routine Immunization Management System—managed by the Child Health Division of the Ministry). At the outset, this division agreed to the rationale of integration proposed by the NRHM Mission Director and participated in the multiple rounds of discussions to integrate the two data collection formats (EPI and HMIS). After this redesign process, new formats were implemented in the states, which contained a unified data set for immunization. However, for this implementation to succeed, it required the national Child Health Division officials to instruct their respective district and facility staff to 'switch off' the RIMS, and use only the new format in the new software provided. However, these instructions were never clearly articulated and RIMS lingered on in different ways in the states. The reasons for its persistence are unclear, but largely related to the immunization programme managers' perceptions that HMIS data would be less reliable, and that they would lose control over data that highlights their achievements. Whatever the perception, the persistence of RIMS led to serious ambiguities for the field staff about which data collection form they should fill, and programme managers at the district and state levels were confused about which data (RIMS or HMIS) was 'official'. These ambiguities led to the integration effort largely failing, attributed to the inability to effectively coordinate the *implementation logics* of the two programmes, thus demonstrating that integration is not only an issue of design (as the *logic of building data integrity in design* was by and large successful), but requires consistent nurturing and skilful navigation through the various implementation complexities that may arise.

Our third example from India, a detailed case study of the Tamil Nadu experience (Case Study 4.1), primarily illustrates fragmentation at the level of the state health information architecture. It shows this fragmentation to be a product of history, determined by whom the systems were developed for, for what objectives, the technical models chosen, and the institutional conditions, such as the dominance of the statistician cadre and the institutionalized power bases. Navigating through these fragmentation challenges was a long, drawn-out process; in this case, about two years. Even after this complex navigation and sensitive design of the integration solution, there were extreme challenges experienced during its implementation. The integration model needed to be resilient against ongoing shocks and disruptions, such as the departure of the champion; however, it failed to withstand these shocks and was terminated, and not only for technical reasons.

(continued on page 84)

Case Study 4.1 Tamil Nadu, India

Tamil Nadu, a southern state in India, has historically been very progressive with respect to its public health reforms, including the use of ICT applications to support these reforms. However, their long history of engagement with healthcare ICT has, at times, diminished the focus on health, with comparable emphasis not given to the health logic of using information for making health service delivery improvements. Since various ICT initiatives had already taken root in the state, there was a reluctance in the state to accept the new development that came with NRHM reforms and that emphasized decentralization and strengthening of the public health focus. Furthermore, there existed a strong cadre of statisticians in the state, who showed a deep sense of ownership of their respective existing systems and the data geared towards central reporting. A state-level official once stated facetiously, 'In this state, we have too many statisticians and computers, so change is complicated'. The strong existing institutional and technical legacies were difficult to dislodge.

The state had had multiple information and communications technologies (ICT) solutions from different vendors. Some of these included:

Primary Health Centre Online System

This was a web-based system built by a leading software vendor in the country, using Microsoft ASP.net and MySQL (Structured Query Language) as the backend platform. This system was designed to collect aggregated area service data from all primary health centres (PHCs) in the state. While the system provided simple user screens for data entry, replicating all paper forms, it did not offer the end user with the flexibility of adding, deleting, or modifying data elements. The system was primarily designed towards automating the existing reporting system and did not provide functionalities towards the generation of indicators for analysis. Furthermore, the system was limited on interoperability, incapable of generating and uploading reports into the national web portal.

Institutional Service Monitoring Report

The Institutional Service Monitoring Report (ISMR), developed in 1999 in association with DANIDA (Danish International Development Agency), used an optical marker reader (OMR) sheet for data collection, and continued until 2008 despite the introduction of the new PHC Online system.

Monthly PHC performance data—outpatients, inpatients, deliveries, staff strength, lab services, and others—were collected from the PHCs using the OMR sheet, which was then transmitted to the state level through the district-level systems. At the state level, these sheets were scanned by an OMR machine reader and output tables generated. Because the design was hardcoded to sheets, this system was also incapable of providing national-level reports, or carrying out indicator-wise analysis.

Pregnancy and Infant Cohort Monitoring System of Tamilnadu

The Pregnancy and Infant Cohort Monitoring System (PICMS) was designed as a web-based system to track individual beneficiaries (pregnant women and infants) enrolled for the antenatal and immunization programmes, respectively. PICMS was designed to help the field nurses (called ANMs—auxiliary nurse midwife) in providing outreach activities. It had a rigid design, was centrally controlled, and relied on the developer's intervention to make any changes. This name-based system was not integrated with the facility aggregate system, and functioned as a stand-alone, even though nearly more than 60 per cent of the name-based data was required for the facility reports. Further, it was limited in providing analysis and feedback reports to ANMs, whose functions the system was primarily expected to support.

Hospital Information System in Tamilnadu's public hospitals

This system was an electronic medical record system aimed at providing improved clinical care, and also to provide aggregate summary reports required from the hospital for the state. This application was also developed by the same vendor responsible for the PHC Online system. In contrast to the PHC Online system that was deployed across all PHCs, this system was deployed across the network of district and subdistrict hospitals in the state. However, the data from this system was not included while generating the state statistics for the national portal. State statistics depended largely only on data from the online PHC system. This system also did not capture the data from the over 15 medical college hospitals located across the 30 districts, while handling a significant part of the hospitalization and specialist consultations that happened within the district. The medical colleges had another distinct hospital information system. The private hospitals that were enrolled under the state's publicly financed insurance systems also had their own system, but its data could not be aggregated or compared with hospital data from the other systems.

There were various other systems too. Despite this, obtaining an overall view of health status was difficult, since each system was stand-alone, controlled by different groups, and run on different platforms. While the national HMIS reforms announced in 2008 required all states to upload their monthly district-wise performance onto a national online web portal, the various systems together were unable to provide this required report. Towards national compliance, the staff had to enter the district-level data manually into the portal. The existing systems, based on their institutional and technical legacies, continued to live and support their limited constituencies primarily towards statistical reporting. Even by combining all data from the different systems, nearly 10 per cent of the data required to generate reports for the national level was missing.

The head of the state health society (called the Mission Director NHM), who was in charge during what we termed the second phase of the national reforms process (see the Odisha case study, Chapter 3) was a visionary and extremely committed to strengthening public health related analysis in the state. Despite the complex history of IT systems in the state, she slowly, over two years, tried to negotiate with the different constituencies for an incremental strategy for integration. She asked for demonstrations of the DHIS 2 software, and saw its potential as an integration tool through the inscribed features of flexibility, end user control, open source, data analysis, and visualization including geographic information system (GIS). After multiple meetings involving the different stakeholders, the forms were revised and implemented for DHIS 2, which served as the 'integration and analysis' tool for the state.

The integration model was that the PHC Online system would continue to be used to collect the facility-level data, which would be exported into the DHIS 2 using XML data standards. The DHIS 2 would perform three key functions: (i) serve as the district repository of data; (ii) generate the national-level reports, and upload those into the national web portal; and (iii) enable district-level analysis, and provide feedback reports to peripheral institutions in the district. Simultaneously, it was agreed that the ISMR would be discontinued, but the PICMS would continue, potentially to be integrated in the future. Following this decision, the DHIS 2 technical team worked with the state and the software vendor to create a software bridge to enable data transfer from the PHC Online system to DHIS 2, and used it to transfer all legacy data from 2010. In addition, data entry screens covering the missing data elements (required for the national reports) were created in the DHIS 2 to enable direct data entry. The national-level reports could now be generated and uploaded in the national portal, and analytical reports sent to levels below and discussed over video-conference meetings. To enable institutional capabilities to support this new integration model, a team of five state-level master trainers was created, who further provided capacity support to the district teams.

However, soon the Mission Director was transferred to another position, and gradually the integration model that was developing with considerable success eroded away, and finally stopped. This happened in parallel with the loss of emphasis on district-level plans and decentralization at the national level. Morever, the cascade model of training adopted by the state team had taken longer than expected to reach the peripheral workers and they had therefore not experienced the limited gains that were possible from the new approach, and felt little sense of loss when it was withdrawn. There was the need for the mid-level managers to own the integration solution, and defend it, if sustainability was to be achieved. This did not happen.

Moving on from national and state levels, in Case Study 4.2, the fourth example from India that we present, is a description of a system-level integration effort of an electronic medical record (EMR) system with a state HMIS application hosting population aggregate data.

4.3.2 Learnings from the case studies

Through the Tamil Nadu and Himachal examples illustrated in Case Studies 4.1 and 4.2, we have tried to illustrate the various logics that drive integration efforts, ranging from concerns of data, multiplicity of systems, prevalent work-related inefficiencies, building national compliances and strengthening support, and the need to use data. These concerns are a product of history, institutional conditions, power and politics, donor imperatives, technical design issues, and the direction of vendor efforts. Addressing them takes a long time to navigate technically and institutionally, and imparts a continued fragility to the process, often not taking firm root within the governmental systems.

The data exchange module from Himachal provides learning on how to approach integration across systems. A key message is to make the respective systems work first, and then—incrementally and in a bottom-up manner—get the exchange functionality to work and gradually add to it layers of sophistication. In many integration efforts across systems, we find that while the exchange module is being developed, the basic systems from which the data exchange has to be enabled are not up to the mark. An alternative approach to

Case Study 4.2 Integrating EMR data to population aggregates: Himachal Pradesh, India

In Chapter 3, we described the case study of a hospital information system from the state of Himachal Pradesh in India. In this part, we discuss one aspect of the case concerning efforts to take the patient-level data from the hospital system, aggregate it, and export that to the state HMIS application in DHIS 2, in order to develop population-based aggregated reports and indicators. Building such an integration is at the core of the HIE architecture, and many papers and conferences have been discussing it, but on a practical level it has been hard to achieve globally.

The hospital information system developed for the state included a data exchange module, which does the task of aggregating name-based data from the OpenMRS-based application from the hospital and exporting it to the DHIS 2 platform, and gives the ability to create indicators and present them in any type of output required by the state. The architecture adopted is one where the patient-based data gets retained in the hospital server, and only the aggregated data is moved to the state server. This module was developed using the initially WHO-promoted standard SDMX.HD (Statistical Data and Metadata Exchange. Health Domain). Data exchanged included all metadata (data elements and facilities), which were synchronized, taking DHIS as the base and then aggregated and exchanged on periodic basis. The exchanged reports included those for national disease programmes, disease profiles for the population, stocks, and inventory reports.

The hospital information system did not capture basic administrative data such as numbers of sanctioned and available functional beds, and the same for numbers of doctors, specialists, and nurses. Such aggregate and 'semi-permanent' data was stored in the DHIS 2 along with population figures, so that these would serve as denominators, while the numerators would come as the aggregates created from the patient records, and together indicators such as admissions by outpatient departments, average length of stay, and others are calculated.

Designing and implementing the data exchange module was a tremendous challenge. Technically, creating the data transfer required writing hundreds of queries to aggregate and push each data element into DHIS 2. After the module was developed and deployed with the overall hospital information system, data exchange was initially done manually, where a hospital staff member had to activate the exchange module to enable the transfer.

> When even this was not done regularly, HISP India automated this process so that at a fixed time daily, the data would be 'synced'. This too was problematic, because of the intermittent and unreliable internet and power supply. Regardless of these limitations, the exchange process is now operational across all 20 hospitals in the state.

imposing a top-down design is to slowly build on what is working or making the basic pieces work, before adding layers of sophistication to it.

4.4 The How of Integration: Modern Efforts of the Open Health Information Exchange

4.4.1 What is the Open Health Information Exchange?

The Open Health Information Exchange (OHIE) is a contemporary and modern day architectural solution being promoted in the West, and increasingly in LMICs, to address the fragmentation problem of HIS. This signifies a shift wherein the national HMIS begins to be based on the electronic health records, in contrast to the earlier systems where they were based on aggregate reports drawn from the primary care providers' recording registers.

A health information exchange (HIE) represents an architecture or framework, driven by a global community of practice, which seeks to make the sharing of health data across information systems possible. Like a universal translator, an HIE normalizes data and secures the transmission of health information throughout databases, between facilities, and across regions or countries.

This HIE architecture being implemented through the Open Health Information Exchange (OpenHIE) framework (https://ohie.org), comprising of six open source software components, all interacting/interoperating to ensure that health information from various points of service applications is gathered into a unified person-centric medical record. To accomplish this, the exchange normalizes the context in which health information is created across four dimensions: (i) who received the health services; (ii) who provided those services; (iii) where they received the services; and (iv) what specific care they received. By focusing on the four Ws—Whom for, Whom by, Where, and What—of a patient's health visit, the OpenHIE seeks to bring relevant information directly to the point of care to help enhance decision-making; improve the quality, safety and continuity of care; and use information to improve population health. Figure 4.1 represents the proposed architecture underlying the OHIE.

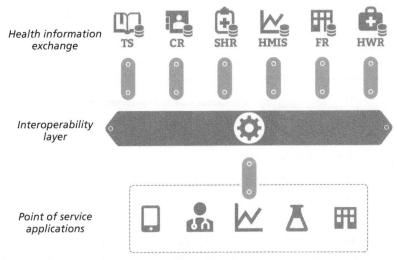

Fig. 4.1 The OpenHIE architecture framework (TS = tracking service; CR = client registry; SHR = shared health record; HMIS = health management information system; FR = facility registry; HWR = health worker registry).

Reproduced with permission from OpenHIE, *Architecture Framework*, OpenHIE: an Open Health Information Exchange Community, Copyright © 2015 OpenHIE. Available from https://ohie.org/#arch, accessed 22nd Jul. 2015.

The figure above sets out the relationship between the different components. We give below a brief definition of each of these components.

Health information exchange

◆ A *terminology service* (TS) serves as a central authority to uniquely identify the clinical activities that occur within the care delivery process by maintaining a terminology set mapped to international standards such as ICO10, LOINC, SNOMED, and others.*Note:* A data and indicator dictionary, which manages metadata important for public health is, so far, not a defined subset of the TS. Or rather, this dictionary is a component that needs to be developed in a way to ensure compatibility with the TS—this would be important in indicating the 'What'? in public health HIS.

◆ An *enterprise master patient index* (EMPI), or *client registry* (CR) manages the unique identity of citizens receiving health services within the country—'For whom'?

◆ A *shared health record* (SHR) is a repository containing the normalized version of content created within the community, after being validated against each of the previous registries. It is a collection of person-centric records for patients with information in the exchange.

+ A *health management information system* (HMIS) stores and manages aggregate data from multiple facilities, health programmes and services, and other data sources. Many of the data sources are paper-based in LMICs, but are increasingly being computerized. The aim of the HMIS is to facilitate data analysis with the goal of improving the quality of health services.

+ A health *facility registry* (FR) serves as a central authority to uniquely identify all places where health services are administered within the country—'Where'?

+ A *health worker registry* (HWR) is the central authority for maintaining the unique identities of health providers within the country—'By whom'?

Health interoperability layer

A health interoperability layer receives all communications from point of service applications within a health geography, and orchestrates message processing among the point of service applications and the hosted infrastructure elements.

Point of service applications

Point of service applications, such as the OpenMRS electronic medical records system and the RapidSMS mHealth application, are to be used by clinicians and by community health workers to access and update a patient's person-centric shared health information and to record healthcare transactions. Countries would have specific applications (e.g. DHIS 2) that serve the roles of the HMIS and FR.

The above-described architecture is expected to solve the technical problems of interoperability. We see here a conscious effort to identify all the components that need to synchronize for interoperability and to suggest a way of inter-relations.

However deceptively easy this architecture may appear on paper, it has been extremely difficult to achieve in practice. It typifies the wickedness of the integration problem in all its facets. We illustrate this through an empirical example from a high-profile initiative in Rwanda (Case Study 4.3), which was one of the pioneering efforts to implement the HIE concept in a LMIC context.

4.4.2 Learnings from the case study

Many nations, including Bangladesh and Phillipines, now seek to replicate the 'Rwanda model'. This case study should, at the very least, point out the challenges and the significant learning curve that is involved.

There are extreme challenges in building an appropriate infrastructure, and a design which is frugal and incremental may be more feasible than one

Case Study 4.3 The Rwanda Health Information Exchange

The Rwanda Health Information Exchange (RHIE) represents a national-level effort of the Rwandan government to promote the creation of a large-scale infrastructure which can potentially drive the generation and use of big and integrated data for health. The objective of the RHIE is to collect and aggregate health data consistently and then promote its broad collaborative reuse by patients, providers, and organizational decision makers. The RHIE represents one of the world's first effort towards a HIE in a LMIC context which has the support of multiple global and national agencies including PEPFAR, CDC, and the Reigenstrief Institute, United States. The RHIE project started in March 2012 within one district (covering 14 health centres and one referral hospital) and focused only on the maternal health programme, a priority area for the Ministry of Health. The aim was to gradually integrate other health programmes into the RHIE framework, and scale on geography.

An evaluation of the RHIE carried out in 2014 identified significant governance challenges. While there were a number of bilateral agreements between various providers, an overall vision, coordination, and its mechanisms were limited. Hampering this coordination was the fact that partners were located in different time-zones, and the reliance on electronic means of communication was ineffective due to the challenges of internet connectivity and reliable power supply in the clinics. Discussions often took place along disciplinary lines with the medicine or IT team seldom talking to each other, and this limited the building of an overall vision. Not enough time was allocated for local capacity and ownership building (Catalani *et al.* 2014). Analysis of data of pregnant women between the HMIS and HIE revealed that more referrals were reported through the HMIS, as also was the case for registrations of antenatal clinics. Evaluation points to the significant challenges that a relatively sophisticated LMIC faces in establishing an appropriate infrastructure to support something as complex as a HIE. A key challenge is to create effective governance mechanisms when stakeholders are multiple, spanning different disciplinary boundaries, and are globally dispersed, relying on electronic communication for coordination. Impacts to date after four years have been limited, with clinicians still preferring to use paper, and no significant impacts been noted on health outcomes. While scalability was a desired end, after about three years and significant resources being invested, the RHIE has not expanded beyond the 14 clinics and one health programme it had started with. On the contrary, the process has scaled down.

which is complex and driven from the top-down. Even in the current set-up of the Rwanda architecture, the incremental approach to the development of a facility register has turned out to be more viable than the top-down approach. The challenges involved in developing and maintaining a register that provides the identification and registration of changes in facilities and their services are bottom-up processes better administered through a live facility-based HMIS reporting system, where changes are continuously reflected more easily than in a stand-alone system. As Rwanda has implemented a best practice cloud-based HMIS system on the DHIS 2 platform, the facility register is already generated and continuously updated within the routine reporting system. The HMIS system will therefore at any point in time have the best updated and authoritative list of facilities. The solution has been that the HMIS and DHIS 2 systems will update the facility register, which is part of the 'Rwanda architecture'; in fact, every five minutes. The problem is that the architecture approach has led to more 'moving parts' and systems to maintain. Furthermore, there are significant challenges in enabling the use of data, and in managing the transition from a paper-based to a complex electronic system, as in the case of the Rwanda architecture. Especially relevant are the challenges clinicians experience in moving over to such an electronic system from their existing manual ones, and these have been difficult to overcome.

4.5 Contemporary Global Integration Priorities and Approaches to Address Them

In this section, we discuss key reform priorities efforts identified by the Global Fund towards strengthening national HMIS within an integrated framework in various high impact countries. These priority areas are now summarized.

4.5.1 Integration of parallel systems into the national health management information system

A key priority is to integrate systems for monitoring the control of HIV/AIDS, tuberculosis (TB), and malaria—IDSR and also EPI, and MCH—into national reporting systems. Strong vertical organizations tend to maintain their own systems, because they feel they can better control their own resources, or only due to legacy. This integration will involve convincing vertical programmes that they would lose none of the current functionalities they enjoy, and that they would benefit from integration based on central repository-based approaches.

4.5.2 **Integrating community health data with the national health management information system**

Community-based data is an important foundation of the health system and most often not well integrated into facility-based reporting systems. This leads to omission of vital information regarding the health status of the population and its follow-up needs. Integrating community-based data, also involving technologies such as mobiles and tablets, is a priority.

4.5.3 **Developing standardized dashboards linked to guidance and training material**

'Dashboards' are identified as a user-friendly way to display integrated information tailored to specific users' needs, which is stored and managed in a data repository, as is in DHIS 2.The aims are to develop (a) templates for dashboards for the different programme areas and for management and M&E; and (b) develop guidelines for the use and sharing of these templates; and (c) develop online demonstration databases where countries can see and learn how to implement the dashboards. The guidelines include suggested naming conventions and standards for indicators and data elements which users will be advised to follow.

4.5.4 **Integrating patient-based and aggregate data to support continuity of care**

Designing systems to support tracking of patients over time to follow them through the cascade of care. This is relevant for many diseases, especially chronic or long-term conditions such as HIV, TB, or programmes like pregnancy and immunization which involve time cycles; for example, the tracking of pregnant women from antenatal care follow-ups through to delivery and postnatal care, and, as a next step, to include infants through immunizations and nutrition services. If a pregnant woman is HIV positive, she should also be tracked across the HIV cascade of care into antiretroviral therapy and its treatment retention.

4.5.5 **Developing and implementing case-based mortality reporting**

Mortality reporting from hospitals has the potential to provide valuable quality information without having to achieve completeness in terms of population covered. Integrating mortality reporting from hospitals with national HMIS, and its standardization based on the International Classification of Diseases (ICD) codes is a global priority.

The WHO has developed a module for ICD10 mortality reporting using the DHIS 2 platform to target resource constrained contexts, which is now being tested in Ghana. It includes a simplified list of 116 diseases, as well as a dictionary of about 6000 diagnoses as a drop down list. As a next step, the WHO team is planning to link the module to an international software (IRIS) used for providing the full correct ICD10 codes.

4.5.6 Developing and implementing tracking systems for case-based disease surveillance

The Ebola crisis has demonstrated the need for case-based disease surveillance and for its integration with the overall HMIS. The Integrated Disease Surveillance and Response programme (IDSR) is, typically, poorly integrated with the national HIS in most countries, and requires the use of case-based tracking systems also based on Android devices for IDSR reporting as an integrated part of the national system.

4.5.7 Developing and implementing tracking systems for case-based malaria control

Malaria pre-elimination requires case-based control. For each case, certain actions are carried out and data is collected. Android-based apps for handheld devices make it possible to use tracking-based systems on mobile phones to support case-based malaria control. These use GPS and plotting of x, y coordinates, and are linked to a GIS. Such Android apps can be used for both general and specific uses, for example, for IDSR, TB, and mortality reporting.

4.5.8 Integrating logistics and drug management in district health information systems and health management information systems

Several countries are using reporting systems to capture some level of commodity/stock availability, varying from stockouts of tracer drugs to more elaborate stock management at facility level. Cold chain management is another application area in logistics management, which provides added value when linked with routine immunization service data, to match demand and supply. Further innovation and standardization of approaches is needed for: integration of specialized logistic management information systems (LMIS) with the national HMIS reporting systems; developing improved visualizations combining service and logistics/stock data; basic stock management at facility levels; and for the use of mobile clients to improve stock reporting and notifications/alerts.

4.5.9 **Developing a facility register combined with an infrastructure dashboard and access system**

The facility register—or Master Facility List—is a key component of this integration work (as shown in Fig. 4.2). To provide access for other systems to the same facility register through the web API (Application Programming Interface) in a standardized way (as in OpenHIE) is a centrally required functionality. Facility infrastructure systems covering resources and services are easily developed using facility register access and information, and are now given high priority in future global health.

The Global Fund has identified the DHIS 2 as an open source data warehouse (http://www.dhis2.org) to serve as a national reference application to support these various integration efforts for both aggregate and case-based reporting.

Indonesia is one of the countries where several of the above integration efforts are currently being implemented as a coordinated effort of various actors, involving the Global Fund, government, University of Oslo, University of Gadjah Madah, HISP India, HISP Vietnam, and others, whose parallel systems are being integrated by transferring key aggregate data from the individual systems to the data warehouse, which again feeds the dashboard. The architecture in the making is presented in Figure 4.2.

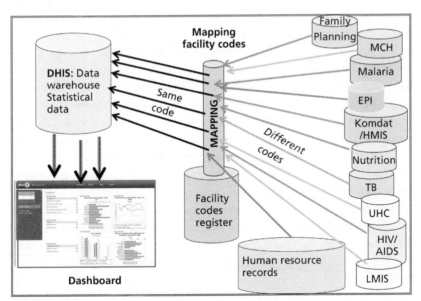

Fig. 4.2 Integration of parallel systems in Indonesia. The health facility register is mapping the different codes for facilities used by the systems so that data can be shared.

In Indonesia, as will be the case for many countries, most of the parallel systems are using their own codes for the health facilities. In order to be able to share facility-based data, it is therefore necessary to map the different codes used for the same facility into one unique ID. The health facility register, as shown in the figure, is maintaining a table of all codes used by the different systems and maps them into the correct facility, so that the data warehouse can combine data from the the different systems that have data on the same facility. We see that several of the priorities listed by the Global Fund are combined into these efforts; integrating parallel systems, such as HIV/AIDS, malaria, as well as also logistics systems (LMIS). In addition, integration with the universal health coverage insurance system is targeted in this effort. We also see that once data is being integrated in the data warehouse for statistical data, the dashboards are relatively easy to design and develop.

4.6 **The Way Forward: Informed by an Expanded PHI Approach**

The discussions around the challenges of integration, illustrated through different case studies, clearly demonstrates that integration is a wicked problem, and not one permitting any easy, short-term solutions. Sometimes, as the case studies from India showed, there are deep-rooted institutional and reporting logics underlying health programmes, which are often intractable, and which makes integration not possible through simple managerialist approaches of getting people around the table to talk consensus. The logic of design is also different from that of implementation. A different set of actors get involved in the field, and the time taken to achieve linkages is far more than what project time schedules tend to allow. State-sponsored integration efforts are usually championed by enlightened bureaucrats, who unfortunately do not stay long enough in the position to institutionalize the change. They have to deal with a historical legacy of many, many systems that have become embedded over decades of projects. Uprooting them requires more than rational arguments of efficiencies and health improvements. One strategy to deal with this problem is an incremental approach like dashboards overlaid on existing systems, which do not politically disturb existing power–information configurations. The value they add through new features like attractive analysis and dashboards that help visualization are more acceptable. This then provides a point of entry for further rationalization and integration efforts. OpenHIE frameworks for integration are complex, top-down architectures, which are difficult to scale. There are also dire implementation challenges. This is illustrated in the Rwanda case study.

So, how does the Expanded PHI approach that we are advocating in this book help to try to find at least partial solutions to these challenges? We draw upon some of the design principles articulated in Chapter 2 to develop implications for approaching this integration.

4.6.1 Understanding the different whys and wherefores of integration

More often than not, integration efforts are driven by a technical logic, with the underlying assumption being that new and more technologies will address existing problems. This is a thoroughly inadequate approach, as firstly, we address the wrong problem, and secondly, this may introduce new problems because of the technological interventions which do not support the underlying and multiple logics. These logics come from the nature of the health programme, the particular institutions involved, choices and influences in design, and the problems and perceptions of those involved in implementation. Understanding the underlying logics which have contributed to the fragmentation, and of the interested stakeholders, would help evolve a more effective overall approach that covers technical, institutional, human, and political considerations. This approach would help to further define the operational plan for the integration. Understanding the different whys and wherefores requires by design a multidisciplinary perspective which brings in inputs from technology, public health, management, sociology, implementation, and others. Otherwise, we get straitjacketed to a merely technical solution, and an information system that is separated from the domain and its surrounding context.

4.6.2 Adopting evolutionary approaches for flexible integration

Building integration as a one-stop solution will necessarily be inadequate, as this is an evolving problem, where new problems and solutions will continuously come into play. Braa and Sahay (2012) have argued that instead of treating architectures as a finished product and as a noun, it may be more effectively treated as a verb—'architecting'. It is an architecture which is always evolving, and at any point will be shaped by incomplete knowledge, as we never know for sure what the future holds. Similarly, integration may be better understood as 'integrating', accepting that it is always a work in process, and can serve as a roadmap for good design. This perspective will help enable design choices that are geared towards flexibility, user control, and avoiding choices which could preclude future opportunities which we currently do not know about. The use of open source platforms and standards becomes key to this approach, as it does not harbour restrictions and licence encumbrances.

4.6.3 **Adopting bottom-up design supported by good governance for integration**

Top-down, centralized design of health architectures has proven to be a recipe for failure, even in rich countries. In LMICs, where resources and expertise are far more limited, attempting to replicate such megalomaniac design blueprints is a far more utopian endeavour. The principle of 'context matters' requires the development of more locally sensitive design approaches. These are not matters of technology 'transfer and replication', but those of sensitive cultivation in context. The work of AEHIN (Asia E-Health Information Network) is inspirational in this regard. In this example, the HIE architecture was a starting point, which has to be adapted to the Asian context, by enabling networks of people from respective countries to participate and be engaged in developing locally relevant solutions. AEHIN also advocates for strong governance mechanisms to be established at the 'top' to ensure an appropriate high-level political body that can evaluate different choices, and provide directions and norms to the management layer to take responsibility for implementation. This combining of good governance at the top, and bottom-up-driven design, may help to try and avoid the problems of top-down, person-driven systems. It would also ensure that the good design practices developed through everyday work can be scaled up to appropriate levels.

4.6.4 **Allowing for time to embed integration solutions**

Integration, by its socio-technical nature, requires significant time to be embedded in institutional settings. The short timeframe project frameworks, as is normally the case of externally funded initiatives, are in deep tension with the time required for such integration to take firm root and be resilient. Even where promising, efforts would not survive beyond the pilot stage—a situation derisively referred to as 'pilotitis'. However, we are not making a case for starting on scale—but for a phased approach. Time is required to get the tools right and build up capacity to implement. Time is also required to allow for users to get familiar with the new ways of working entailed by the integrated solution, and gradually be able to see the added value it brings. Only with this deeper use can new solutions take root, and acquire resilience to endure over time. Expecting short-term solutions, even if it involves more modern technologies, we argue is the wrong way to approach this problem.

4.7 **Conclusions**

This chapter has taken up the wicked and all-pervasive problem of fragmentation, and examined why integration solutions have been difficult to come to institutional fruition. Some of the different challenges and solutions faced have been discussed through empirical examples the authors have been engaged with over the years. Some contemporary approaches such as the HIE have been discussed, emphasizing the problems of centralized and complex architectures. Some contemporary integration priorities identified by Global Fund have been discussed, all of which are currently works in progress, which we are following up on and will add to our learnings. Finally, drawing from the design principles of the Expanded EPI, four metalevel learnings are identified to guide such integration efforts, viz. understanding the multiple logics of the systems requiring integration; adopting an evolutionary and dynamic approach in contrast to a one-time fixed one; adopting a bottom-up approach supported by visionary and strong governance support from above; and, finally providing adequate time for embedding integration solutions.

4.8 **References**

Braa, J. and Sahay, S. (2012). *Integrated Health Information Architecture: Power to the Users: Design, Development and Use*. Matrix Publishers, New Delhi, India.

Catalani, C., Hoth, A., Seymour, D., Nelson, T., Kayigamba, F., Gakuba, R. (2014). Best Practices for Building an Integrated National Health Information System: Rwanda. GHF2014, Innovation and Technologies, Research project [Online]. Available at: http://ghf.g2hp.net/2014/02/25/best-practices-for-building-an-integrated-national-health-information-system-rwanda/ [Last accessed 1 October 2015].

Health Metrics Network (2008). *Health Metrics Network, Framework and Standards for the Development of Country Health Information Systems*. World Health Organization. Available at: http://apps.who.int/iris/bitstream/10665/43872/1/9789241595940_eng.pdf

The World Bank (2015). Health, Nutrition and Population Data and Statistics. Corporate and Global Results Monitoring. [Online] Available at: http://datatopics.worldbank.org/hnp/strategy [Last accessed 1 October 2015].

WHO (2005). Fifty-Eighth World Health Assembly—Resolutions And Decisions Annex. [Online]. Available at: http://apps.who.int/gb/ebwha/pdf_files/WHA58-REC1/english/A58_2005_REC1-en.pdf [Last accessed 1 October 2015].

WHO (2013). Sixty-Sixth World Health Assembly—eHealth standardization and interoperability. [Online]. Available at: http://www.who.int/ehealth/events/wha66_r24-en.pdf [Last accessed 1 October 2015].

World Summit on Information Society declaration (2003). Plan of Action. Document WSIS-03/GENEVA/DOC/5-E, [Online] Available at: http://www.itu.int/dms_pub/itu-s/md/03/wsis/doc/S03-WSIS-DOC-0005!!PDF-E.pdf [Last accessed 1 October 2015].

Chapter 5

Decentralized Information Use: Are The Cloud and Big Data Supporting This?

5.1 The Cloud, Big Data, and Data Analytics

For many, the cloud offers the 'new dawn' for low and middle-income countries (LMICs), bringing in opportunities for creating national databases, modernization of infrastructure, opportunities for enterprise, and various other trappings of modernity. Many have described the cloud as the platform for LMICs to leapfrog the digital divide. Discussions on 'big data' have become almost synonymous with discussions of the cloud because by sheer nature of its volume and diversity, big data could be better harnessed by the cloud than by traditional computing infrastructure. However, as we move data (big or small) towards the cloud, we run the risk of being distanced from the local information infrastructure in terms of access and ownership, and face arguments of being less grounded for reasons of relevance, particularity, as well as data sovereignty. These opposing tendencies are best conceptualized in dialectic terms where a move in one direction inherently contradicts and undermines the other—the stronger the movement to the cloud, the greater is the sense of loss of the local infrastructure and ownership. In a dialectical understanding such contradictions are inevitable, but they also go along with the unity of opposites.

The question this chapter explores is the nature of these contradictory forces around big data and the cloud, and the apparently universal character it imparts to the perceptions of information on one hand and the context-bound and particular character of the production and use of information on the other. This analysis leads to a better understanding of the implications these trends have for decentralization of health systems and health information systems (HIS) that are currently the target of major national, regional, and global reform efforts. Do the cloud and big data represent in themselves sufficient game-changers to help rectify the health systems problems and challenges of the past, such as of fragmentation, or do they create larger problems out of our control?

Before discussing implications of the cloud, it becomes imperative to peel the layers that comprise it, in order to understand its nature and uses.

5.2 **What is Cloud Computing?**

Underneath the cloud are material and commercial components comprised of servers, data centres, networks, and business models which need to be better understood. Cloud computing flows from these developments, and is fast becoming an industry buzzword. As Larry Ellison, CEO of Oracle Corporation, is reported to have said at the Oracle Openworld conference: 'The interesting thing about cloud computing is that we've redefined cloud computing to include everything that we already do'. The danger arising from the ubiquitous use of the term *cloud* is that it gets idolized, and masks the objective and material (technical and commercial) elements of what we are talking about. Furthermore, the work which goes into making these components functional and sustaining them over time, becomes increasingly invisible.

5.2.1 **Defnition and components of cloud computing**

The National Institute of Standards and Technology—NIST—has provided a well-accepted definition of cloud computing (Mell and Grance 2011):

> 'Cloud computing is a model for enabling ubiquitous, convenient, on-demand network access to a shared pool of configurable computing resources (e.g., networks, servers, storage, applications, and services) that can be rapidly provisioned and released with minimal management effort or service provider interaction.' (p. 2)

Based on the NIST guidelines, the essential characteristics, service models, and deployment models are listed as follows:

Essential characteristics

- ◆ On-demand self-service
- ◆ Broad network access
- ◆ Resource pooling
- ◆ Rapid elasticity
- ◆ Measured service

Service models

- ◆ Software as a Service
- ◆ Platform as a Service
- ◆ Infrastructure as a Service
- ◆ Analytics as a Service

Cloud deployment models

- Private cloud
- Community cloud
- Public cloud
- Hybrid cloud

The essential characteristics and service models listed above are further discussed in Chapter 7. Here we briefly discuss the deployment models.

5.2.2 **Deployment models**

Private cloud

The cloud infrastructure is provisioned for exclusive use by a single organization. It may be owned, managed, and operated by the organization, a third party, or some combination, and it may exist on or off premises.

Community cloud

The cloud infrastructure is provisioned for exclusive use by a specific community of consumers from organizations that have shared concerns. It may be owned, managed, and operated by one or more of the organizations in the community, a third party, or some combination of them, and it may exist on or off premises.

Public cloud

The cloud infrastructure is provisioned for open use by the general public. It may be owned, managed, and operated by a business, academic, or government organization, or some combination of them. It exists on the premises of the cloud provider.

Hybrid cloud

The cloud infrastructure is a composition of two or more distinct cloud infrastructures (private, community, or public) that remain unique entities, but are bound together by standardized or proprietary technology that enables data and application portabilities.

5.2.3 **Technical configurations and business models**

Taking these definitions and characteristics as the point of departure, we can infer two key underlying objective elements that define the cloud:

i) The technical configuration
ii) The business model

The technical configuration represents, firstly, the kind of hosting platform, and the different essential characteristics that allow hosting of websites/applications on virtual servers, which pull computing resources from extensive underlying networks of physical web servers shared by multiple users. The business model includes the service model, the type of cloud deployment, and other contractual agreements between the provider, client, and any third party agencies. This includes how the server space is allocated to different users based on the fees paid. Different combinations of the technical configuration and business models can be said to underlie the 'cloud infrastructure'. For example, the state information technology (IT) department of a ministry can run their own data centre and a private cloud, where they offer services for free or at a fee to the health department. Alternatively, there can be a contract where the state gets a third party to host their application on the public cloud, using Linode, at a monthly fee. And, there can be various different combinations of the technical configuration and the business model, making it important for us to be clear about their meaning when the term 'cloud' is used.

While the cloud is seen to be cost-effective and elastic, Vaughan-Nichols (2015) argues that there is nothing like a free lunch, as currency fluctuations (in the USD, Euro, or Norwegian Krone) may suddenly hike up real prices. Recently, the three big public cloud services—Google Cloud Platform, Amazon Web Services, and Microsoft Azure—raised their prices. Azure did so by 13 per cent in the Eurozone and 26 per cent in Australia, as also did Microsoft by 26 per cent. Business models are governed by forces of capitalism, and subject to the necessary influences which come with it. This raises the need to examine alternatives of keeping data in-house where there can be more control over the costs, or use hybrid models of the cloud to hedge risks of global currency fluctuations.

The cloud infrastructure is typically made available to users through the 'service' model which provides for process storage, networks, and fundamental computing resources. It is made operational through an 'outsourcing' model as followed in the general IT software and services area, but with a key difference. Traditional software outsourcing was done from the rich (such as United States and United Kingdom) to the not so rich countries (like India, Vietnam, and China) primarily for cost advantages, and because necessary human resources were not available in-country. Starting from the 1980s, this outsourcing industry has flourished, today becoming a thriving and profit-making one, particularly in countries like India, providing gainful employment to large numbers of people. Interestingly, cloud outsourcing works the other way round, where many LMIC users and governments access cloud hosting service in the rich countries, because they are able to provide the cloud infrastructure at more cost-effective prices and more reliable services than what typically would be provided for by companies from LMICs.

In public health informatics this seems an attractive proposition. One could, for example, use online computing to replace hundreds of offline facility-level installations with one central, online server. This should potentially enable integration and render superfluous to a large extent the problem of end users having to do technical maintenance of local hardware and software. However, as we saw in Chapter 4, the terms at which information is produced, disseminated, and consumed contributes to how it is valued and used. New problems may emerge through the use of central online servers or the use of someone else's infrastructure (such as global companies) through rental agreements. For example, control could shift to large global companies and their affiliates who run the cloud infrastructure, giving them, potentially, control over the data. These issues are part of a spectrum of concerns related to control over information and overlap debates about net neutrality, open data, development, data sovereignty, and similar such issues. In-between these broader questions over the emerging political economy of information, we also discuss the operational aspects of the cloud and big data, and how LMICs are trying alternative models to operationalize them, and what some of the empirical experiences have been.

In summary, we argue that the cloud must be viewed in terms of a confluence of business model and technology, which are, to a certain extent, autonomous with different driving forces but also very much in dialectic relation to one another with respect to nature (power, cooling, green technology, etc.), labour (who does work for whom, and when and who gains value from the work), everyday life (e.g. the actual health consequences to the non-professional 'beneficiary'), and more. Further, the global geo-political-strategic importance of information, surveillance, security, big data, and various other non-economic factors of production are also at play.

While the focus of this chapter is primarily on the cloud, in line with our Expanded PHI approach, we argue that discussions on the cloud are incomplete without discussing big data (what is stored in the cloud) and data analytics capabilities (ability to pull data out of the cloud). These have implications on the institutions and people involved, and their inter-relations. The identified issues around the cloud are explored in the context of these inter-connections.

5.3 Cloud Infrastructure for Health in Low and Middle-Income Countries: Becoming Increasingly 'Autonomous'?

Way back in the 1970s, Langdon Winner coined the term 'autonomous technology' to theorize the relation between technological complexity and control (Winner 1978). As technologies become increasingly complex, and as the locus of control shifts to non-local locations, technology becomes increasingly 'autonomous', taking on a life of its own and thus becoming more difficult to control. As an example, the blinds of the windows in the modern office at the University of Oslo in Norway are controlled by automatic sensors. Depending on the intensity of the sun (or its absence), the movement of the blinds is auto-controlled. From the perspective of an occupant of the office, the technology is becoming increasingly autonomous giving him or her limited control, as compared to earlier when the window could be just manually opened or closed, or the curtains pulled out or in. Now the movement of the blinds is under increasing control of non-local forces, with decreased control of the local actors. The theme of 'autonomous technology' has also been picked up by science fiction novels and characters. *Frankenstein* was perhaps the first of these, representing a creature built by technology turning against its very creator. Now movies and television shows are full of run-away artificial intelligence systems where the robots become autonomous and seek to control and destroy the masters who created them. *The Matrix* trilogy and *I Robot* are perhaps the most successful cinematic examples of this trend in science fiction.

In a much more mundane manner, we see problems of autonomous technology in daily life. An interesting question this raises in the context of HIS in LMICs is whether the cloud and big data have tendencies to take on similar autonomous characteristics, viewed from the perspective of the user or the state in the LMIC, and if so, what are its implications? The technologies of the cloud, big data, and associated analytics are in themselves complex, when combined more so, and are normally under control of multiple non-local agents.

In the following section, we seek to understand the alternative models being used to operationalize these technologies in LMICs.

5.4 **Cloud Infrastructure: Moving from 'Closer to Machine' Applications to Further Away**

The cloud has enabled many national web-based systems in LMICs to become feasible because of the improved network infrastructure. Access has widened with increased geographical coverage of mobile networks, wider spread of mobiles, use of modems, and improvements in computer networks. Improved connectivity within and to other nations has made possible the physical location of servers outside of the Ministries of Health, co-located within private data centres such as internet service providers, purpose-built national data centres, and various global providers. Ironically, these providers may utilize helpdesk and systems admin support through outsourcing arrangements in developing countries like India. Physical infrastructure would tend to be located in the North, which is probably a question of trust and regulation. If these global providers could create data centres in other countries at lower costs, they probably would. But these may not sell as well as having data in the more 'trusted' locations of New York, London, or Tokyo.

Outsourcing of software development and services has been widely studied by information systems researchers, especially over the last two decades. After the initial excitement of the business, financial, and employment opportunities generated in the early 1980s and 1990s, researchers have studied the extreme difficulties in making these relationships work over time. For example Sahay *et al.* (2003), based on longitudinal, empirical studies involving about a dozen countries, and interviews with more than 500 managers, conceptualized outsourcing as an evolving relationship which needs to be nurtured over time. These relationships are shaped by conditions of culture, time and space, communication styles, power and politics, knowledge asymmetries, and various other factors. In their study, they narrate the story of a relationship between an English and an Indian firm engaged in an outsourcing arrangement. The English firm is a client whose central concern is presented as how to impose the 'English way' of working on their Indian partners. This is met with the expected resistance from the Indians, leading to the ultimate breakdown of the relationship. In a less typical study, Silva (2002) describes a case of a reverse arrangement, where the Guatemalan Ministry of Health outsources the development of a hospital administration system to a consultancy company. Silva explicitly introduces the dimension of power into his analysis in understanding whether the arrangement worked or not.

The outsourcing of cloud services from LMICs to rich countries can be seen to also follow a similar trajectory. In the initial stages, there is widespread excitement as it helps to 'black-box' the technological concerns at more competitive prices. What is being outsourced here is just the physical hosting of data and applications in a distant and more effective infrastructure. The need for human and institutional interaction is relatively limited in these 'closer to machine' applications. However, as these relationships mature, and clients look for more advanced services such as data analytics using the data stored in the cloud, or more sophisticated services around optimization of databases and applications, one can expect the need for more human interactions. These will then come with the usual challenges that such interactions involve, especially concerning governance of cloud-based relationships. In Chapter 7 we argue that such 'high end' services related to the governance of more complex information systems will, as a rule, not be possible to 'black-box' and outsource.

Whereas currently the characteristics of cloud are broadly understood, governance of cloud services from the client perspective appears to be less so. In a comprehensive review of 25 leading journals, Hoberg *et al.* (2012) reveal that 'no paper could be found which develops or applies a governance framework tailored to the specific challenges users are confronted with when adopting cloud services' (p. 7). These challenges of governance are especially magnified in the context of governments in LMICs, especially concerning regulation of issues of data sovereignty, ownership and access, and of managing knowledge asymmetries.

In section 5.5, we discuss how LMIC governments are trying to leverage cloud infrastructure to operationalize web-based HIS applications, and the challenges they face. Following this, we look at 'further from the machine' applications, where efforts are made to leverage the capabilities of big data analytics based on cloud infrastructure, and the underlying challenges and opportunities.

5.5 Leveraging Cloud Infrastructure: Health Applications in Low and Middle-Income Countries

As web-based applications are becoming increasingly prominent in LMICs, Ministries of Health are being confronted with the question of what are the appropriate models to host these applications and the emerging implications. We begin with a case study from India that examines issues around the operationalization of cloud hosting for the DHIS 2 application across different states in Case Study 5.1, and then in next section, Case Study 5.2 discusses another example from Kenya using deployment of the cloud.

The Kenyan example supports the idea of a professional hosting service provider as an important contributor for the successful implementation of an online system, because the focus could be on ensuring the users' access to the internet and not on the proper functionality of the server and its connectivity. When implementing online web-based systems, the server is extremely critical as it needs to be optimally accessible nearly 100 per cent of the time. The new paradigm of online web-based systems is breaking with the tradition of each organization and ministry having their own computer centre and servers. Implementing systems 'on the web', means that it does not rely on any particular physical location. The new situation following Snowden and the US National Security Agency scandal has rightly put the attention on data security and the need for countries to ensure sovereignty over their own data.

Zimbabwe rolled out DHIS 2 in 2014 and decided to host the server in Ministry of Health building. This had a lot of problems, such as poor conditions in the server room and very poor connectivity to the internet, because

(continued on page 111)

Case Study 5.1 India: The Challenges of Scale

In India, the DHIS 2 has been in use at state level for the last 10 years, and various models of hosting have been tried, with different challenges and solutions. Some of these experiences are now discussed.

Typically, in a small state like Himachal Pradesh with 12 districts covering a population of nearly 20 million, there are in general about 1200 system users, and during the monthly data entry, this volume increases by almost 25 per cent. A state like Maharashtra which has about 35 districts covering a population of about 114 million, the application must support about 3600 users, and roughly 25 per cent more during the peak data entry period.

The average capacity of the server is estimated at 16 to 32 GB RAM, with 16 core CPU, 700 GB HDD, and 1 TB of data transfer per month. This capacity estimation is not done on very professionally defined criteria, but typically follows the principle of 'the higher the capacity, the better', which may not be the most cost-effective solution. HISP India, which manages the servers in many of the states, are also learning by doing, and many mistakes on estimation have been made on the way. From the state's perspective, problems related to inadequate server capacity are often attributed to 'problems in the DHIS 2', often creating a stand-off with each side blaming the other.

In terms of hosting options, some states are using the government data centre which provides services to all government departments, including the health department. Often these IT departments are rather restrictive, providing remote access to only one IP address, limiting who can provide support and from where. Then there are demands for the DHIS 2 supporting organization (in this case HISP India) to provide a security testing certificate whenever a change is made in the source code. Given that this security testing, conducted through the National IT department or a third party certified agency, is a time-consuming process (often taking more than six months) and also expensive (costing about USD 5000 to be borne by HISP India), it has impeded version upgrades and the states have lagged behind in current releases of DHIS 2.

Some states have opted for a third party data hosting centre located within the country, in compliance with state policy that their data should not leave the country. However, they have been struggling with developing appropriate service level agreements (SLAs) with the vendor, and monitoring effective service provision. They also feel they are overcharged.

Some other states have opted for cloud (Linode) hosting, which while being the relatively more inexpensive option of the three, is not acceptable to most states as they perceive that data will be stored in a US server, and thus subject to their laws.

There are other reasons why cloud-based deployment has not picked up across states as was expected initially. While the cloud provides benefits of quick deployment, scalable infrastructure with usage-based pricing, and no upfront hardware and resource costs, there were associated challenges related to infrastructure, user load, and security. Accessing data stored on the server requires a sound internet connection. In addition to contracting and locational issues, there were other problems relating to hard-to-reach physical servers for any type of recovery, and backup services offered only at additional costs. The cloud assumes the existence of good and robust internet infrastructure, which is often not the case in many states, leading to problems with server speed due to slow I/O (input/output) rates, and challenges for users to do data entry or generate reports on the fly. The cloud is also vulnerable to security concerns, since all ports tend to be open to the public, and there is the need to identify and block the unrequired ports. The service provider is expected to provide hardware and locational security, which is not possible to verify. Similarly, operating system security also remains vulnerable to attacks by viruses and hackers. Another minor but troublesome problem is that extending rental agreements for cloud-based servers are through credit card payment, which under the rules is not an option for direct financing by Ministry of Health of Ministry-owned servers.

Through various experiences of learning by doing, HISP India, which operates the servers on which DHIS 2 works, for a number of states, have developed various means to strengthen security, such as updating software regularly, establishing firewalls, and setting up reverse proxy servers which have low memory footprints and are easy to use. Blocking shell access to the box through SSH (secure socket shell) configuration is also an important security mechanism, and configuration options added to the SSHD (solid state hybrid drive) configuration file helps to restart the SSHD server and reload the configuration options. Passwords are stored in encrypted formats as a one-way function, where a lost password can be reset but not recovered. Maintaining access logs and audit trails allows for stronger governance of security. Carrying out third party security certification has also helped enhance the security mechanisms.

Case Study 5.2 Kenya's Challenges with the Cloud: The First National Cloud-based HIS in Africa

In 2011, Kenya was the first country in Africa to implement an online national HIS data warehouse for the universal capture and use of routine data, based on a central server solution. The long-awaited sea cable had arrived in East Africa on the coast in Mombasa, late in 2010. Cables were laid inland to Nairobi, and internet over the mobile network was rapidly covering the country. The rest of inland East Africa, including Rwanda and Uganda, followed over the next couple of years. The implementation in Kenya unfolded differently than in the cases from India, where the system was mostly accessed through fixed internet lines. The implementation in Kenya was solely based on the cloud. While the users accessed the system by the use of modems to the internet over the mobile network, the server for the system itself was hosted by Linode, a cloud service company based in London, following the 'Infrastructure as a Service' model.

Online state-wide installations of the HIS data warehouse using the DHIS 2 platform had been in use in India since 2009 at the state level, but for Africa it was still regarded as impossible to establish an online system with national coverage. Also, in Kenya the initial plan in October 2010 was to combine offline stand-alone installations in districts with poor internet with online systems in districts with good internet. When testing the internet access to the first prototype system in a rural hospital, everything was fine until a power cut occurred, and despite the hospital's generator quickly returning the power, the fixed internet line went down. The conclusion that 'Africa was not yet ready for the internet' was just about to be reached when somebody tested the modem to the mobile internet option and found that it worked well. At that time, modems to the internet had not been regarded as being stable enough for a national production system. However, testing of modem-based internet was quickly carried out around the country and it was found to be good enough. The strategy was then changed from a partly offline to a fully online and cloud-based installation of a web-based data warehouse on the DHIS 2 platform.

Over the next six months, rapid prototyping of the Kenya data warehouse application was carried out, including a lot of development on the software platform itself in order to make it better cope with the new situation of limited internet and a new concept of 'semi-online' deployment. New functionalities were implemented directly on the online server and made available for all users on the spot, which again helped to generate feedback, adjustments, and requirements for new functionalities. User participation and rapid cycles of development were greatly enabled by the new online development environment; and in order to enable users to quickly learn about and start using and testing new functionalities, a 'Facebook Light' was developed as part of the DHIS 2 platform. The system users in Kenya quickly started to communicate, by district or province or nationwide; informing each other about new functionalities, feedback, technical problems, and support.

During the rollout, nearly all data managers raised the issue of internet connectivity costs. This was addressed by the provision of modems and airtime. A further step was the development of an offline data entry capability. The new HTML5 web browser standard allowed for offline data entry, as browsers implementing this standard now include a small database, thus improving the robustness of internet connectivity in rural parts of Kenya. Users capture data offline by using the memory in the browser and upload the data to the server when online. The following message was posted by a user at messaging system after the new feature of offline data capture had been included:

13 September 2011

> Hi, this is wow! I have realized that I can now work with a lot of
> ease without any interruptions from network fluctuations since some of
> us are in the interiors where we have lots of challenges with the
> network. This is so good, a big Thank you ...

The web-based national data warehouse system in Kenya was implemented using the international cloud hosting company Linode, on a server physically located in London. The hosting outside the country's borders has been an issue of concern throughout the process. First, the server and data centre in the Ministry of Health in Kenya could not have been used for the implementation; the internet connection to the Ministry building and the server was very poor, and the server itself was not adequate.

The staff working in the building were also all using their own private modems to access the internet because the fixed internet was poor. Second, in 2013, the hosting was temporarily moved to Safaricom, a Kenyan mobile operator also providing cloud services. However, the services provided by them were inadequate and the system moved back to Linode. It was disappointing that the national hosting company did not have a good enough standard.

there was no dedicated line but only the general line, used by everyone. Capacity to manage the server and ensure power backup 24/7 are other general problems. When countries require servers to be within their national boundaries, this needs to be supported by a national policy to establish quality and secure hosting environments, either in private or governmental data centres.

The recommended approach is to procure such hosting services from external providers, which relieves the Ministry of Health, or the organization, of providing necessary features such as backup electricity solutions, regular data backup, server maintenance and security and reliable internet/network access, all of which are difficult to find within the existing structure of the health system. A typical policy concern is the in-country location of the data storage, but this can be mitigated with special arrangements with the provider, or by using national providers. The problem is that many countries in Africa do not have adequate hosting alternatives in the country.

The following are the generally acknowledged requirements for a hosting environment, or data centre:

i)   Human capacity for server administration and operation. There must be human resources with general skills in server administration and in the specific technologies used for the application providing the services. Examples of such technologies are web servers and database management platforms.

ii) Reliable solutions for automated backups, including local off-server and remote backup.

iii) Stable connectivity and high network bandwidth for traffic to and from the server.

iv) Stable power supply including a backup solution.

v)   Secure environment for the physical server regarding issues such as access, theft, fire, drainage in case of water leakage, and good procedures for cleaning.

vi) An operational disaster recovery plan containing a realistic strategy for making sure that the service will be only suffering short downtimes in the events of hardware failures, network downtime, and more.

vii) Feasible, powerful, and robust hardware.

In many LMICs, ambitious plans to go onto digital platforms must be accompanied by the readiness to invest in such infrastructure. And, it would require professional support from outside government ministries to achieve this.

5.6 **Reflecting on Paradoxes of the Cloud and Local Use of Data**

The rapid scale-up of the internet and the mobile networks, and their combination—viz. the availability of internet over the mobile network—have ensured that health workers and communities, even those in remote rural settings of LMICs, are increasingly familiarized with the internet and will start seeing it as a natural part of their work life. Access to the internet over the mobile network now tends to increase faster and reach wider than even technology-optimistic system developers have been able to anticipate. For example, while assessing a mobile telephone SMS-based disease reporting system (RapidSMS) in the most remote parts of Zimbabwe, it was found that the health workers had switched to using the internet-based service WhatsApp on their personal smart phones instead of using the SMS system on the phones provided by the Ministry of Health, which they found cumbersome. It is a paradox that the implementation of a 'modern' mobile-based reporting system is already bypassed by technological development in such a way that users have already switched to smart phones privately and find it easier to use a cloud-based internet service, even though they have to use their own phones and pay for it themselves.

Thus we are now approaching a new situation where there is access to the internet everywhere, which, in theory, is making 'all the information of the world' available through computers and handheld devices, and providing instant online communication facilities to most people, even, increasingly, the rural poor. The internet revolution thus seems to provide a tremendous potential for public health: through advocacy, dissemination of information and health education, and through involving communities in social media and many other yet to be discovered approaches.

While the space of good usage of the cloud in public health is open, our aims here are more narrow in the sense that we focus on the HIS aspects of the cloud, where we encounter two paradoxes. First, it is a paradox that while the internet revolution has given a large and constantly increasing number of people in LMICs online access to, in principle, an unlimited number of information sources, why then are quality data on the community and health services, which are addressing the needs of public health, still largely of poor quality, paper-based, or in other ways inaccessible due to poor systems and fragmentation? One key concern in this chapter is of how to make PHI fully leverage these new opportunities to make effective and easy to access systems. However, while addressing this topic of making good and locally grounded information systems in the internet age, we meet the other paradox. As we move data and systems from the local computers and hands-on control to the 'internet', or the cloud, which by definition is 'far away', are we not then being distanced from the local, in terms of access and ownership and the particularities and relevance of the local data, as well as data sovereignty?

Assessing the usage of DHIS 2 in remote parts of Kenya, we asked a similar question to a local user; whether he felt that he had less access and control of his own data now, with the data in the cloud, than before, when he had the data on his PC? No, he responded, this is like Facebook, I have access to my own data as well as data from other districts, continuously updated, anytime, and from anywhere. Before, access to data was more difficult as it was inside one computer in the office. And it was difficult to show to others.

The key advantage of having the HIS data in the cloud is that all users from all levels in the hierarchy can access the data. In Kenya, it is even possible for anyone to create their own account and to access the data. Before, in the pre-cloud area, the information officers who controlled the data in the stand-alone computers would have the role of gate keepers and it would be necessary to go through them to get the data. Both because of the de-facto institutional arrangements of giving individuals or the HIS unit the power to control the access to data and the technical difficulties in actually disseminating the data and giving people access, data was hard to get hold of in many places under the pre-internet technological paradigm. Of course, with the internet, control of who gets access to what data will still be there. But since the electronic platform for sharing data has drastically changed, the issue of providing access to the data will have to be debated at a more transparent level as higher level management will have a say, and the general user will demand access. The 'like Facebook' understanding of local information in the cloud, as put forward by the local user in Kenya, is also illustrating that wide user groups would now be more demanding and will know that they should have the right to access their own and also other data in the cloud.

In Chapter 7 we present the case of Ghana (Jolliffe *et al.* 2015), which is demonstrating that moving the data to the cloud led to better access by wide user groups from all levels of the health service. By providing access to the data to more users and wider user groups, increased transparency and use of the data, at least at a basic level, will follow. Increased access and use will generally lead to more feedback, and we may argue, better quality data. In Ghana it is documented that the increased access and use of the data in the new cloud-based system has led to increased data quality.

5.7 Cloud Infrastructure: Leveraging Big Data and Bigger Expectations

Discussions on big data are inevitably intertwined with that of the cloud, as the latter is undoubtedly a driver of big data. Some time back, during a discussion in the Indian Ministry of Health on why there should be national-level storage of individual pregnancy data, the response from the Ministry was 'now servers are so big, we can store all data'—a classical technical solution to an issue related to the public health rationale of the need for the data being collected and acted upon.

Currently, there are various questions on the table on whether and how big data can lead to its improved applications to strengthen health systems and HIS in LMICs. A data revolution, which big data is enabling in health, involves a radical shift in data generation, collection, and use practices from what currently exists. Big data represents large volumes of machine readable data and tools for its analysis, visualization, and interpretation (Pentland *et al.* 2013). Furthermore, big data is characterized by volume and speed, which makes it difficult for an organization to manage using conventional methods and systems (Grossman and Siegel 2014). Big data is termed as the 'new oil' fuelling innovation and the new economy (Beardsley *et al.* 2014). However, this data revolution has not fully arrived, nor is it static; it is continuously in the making, and also evolving. Big data and the cloud carry extreme trappings of modernity, as emphasized by Zuboff's (2014) 'digital declaration'.

> 'When it comes to "big data" and the digital future, we are at the very beginning. Despite the rapid pace of connection and the oceans of data it generates, our societies have yet to determine how all this will be used, to what purpose, and who decides.'

Big data cannot be equated with data revolution, but it is a necessary though not sufficient condition. Big data on its own will not address health systems problems. For the revolution to happen, there are other ingredients that are needed, such as regulation on ethics and legal guidelines, appropriate infrastructure including the cloud, capacities for data analytics, and the political will to bring these different pieces together to create increased sufficiency.

Big data was first defined according to the three Vs of *Volume, Variety*, and *Velocity* (Laney 2001). Later more Vs were added, of which *Veracity* is of particular importance in our context and will be discussed in Chapter 7, as it links directly to the problems of quality of health data. *Volatility* and *Value* are other Vs that have been suggested (Normandeau 2013). Different stakeholders with varying interests seek to leverage the potential of big data to create different kinds of value. Currently, large IT firms, cloud providers, data brokerage firms, and those dealing with analysis of health insurance data dominate this market. A distinction is made between use and exchange value, where the former represents the application of big data for supporting routine operations, and the latter concerns the ability to create intellectual capital to be exploited to generate additional and different forms of value on a continual basis in other settings. A key challenge for LMICs is how to intervene in value flows, and ensure they can generate exchange value for the larger public good.

While bringing data together in a HIS from a variety of sources such as different health programmes and health services, hospitals, health centres, community health workers, finance, drug stocks, labs, human resources, etc., and, for example, adding several layers of maps, we are indeed challenging general techniques for information management. This is what has been referred to as the 'big data' challenge. When integrating multiple and diverse types and sources of data into a data warehouse, we face the challenges of increased Volumes, Velocity, Variety, and Veracity of data.

Furthermore, LMICs use census and survey data, such as district level household surveys, sample registration systems, household and demographic surveys, and various others. For official reporting, governments tend to rely on survey data due to limited trust on routine health management information systems (HMIS) data. Despite the inaccuracies and incompleteness of HMIS data, it is nevertheless one of the most reliable sources of routine data (Keen *et al.* 2013). HMIS data is indeed 'big' in volume, variety, and by default veracity; for example, until 2008, 200,000 public health facilities in India reported on about 3000 data elements monthly. The Tajikistan Ministry of Health reports on about 30,000 data elements from each district on a quarterly basis. However, it is difficult to apply the general modern big data principles of data mining in the context of low-resource settings, where the constraints in themselves add to the 'bigness' of incoming data. Big data in health in LMICs is very different from, for example, the big data handled by Google. Given these vast differences of what is perceived as big data, and the differences in the organizations dealing with the data, Purkayastha and Braa (2013) suggest that 'bigness' of data needs to be defined in terms of an organization's capability to leverage on its potential.

In analysing various national initiatives, many challenges exist in the uptake of systems and the establishment of systematic use. The shift from aggregate monthly data to name and encounter-based data hosted on the cloud could potentially contribute to a data revolution in terms of volume and velocity. However, achieving the stage of effective use is a complex and long-term endeavour, also involving other technologies and capacities. An archetypical example is the often-cited case of Google Flu Trends, which is a web service operated by Google since 2008. This provides estimates of influenza activity for more than 25 countries by aggregating Google search queries. The idea behind this is the monitoring of millions of users' health tracking behaviours online, to detect the presence of flu-like illness in a population (identified by the internet protocol (IP) address of each search). Google Flu Trends compares these findings to a historic baseline level of influenza activity (based on 50 million queries entered weekly in the United States between 2003 and 2008) for its corresponding region and then reports the activity level as either minimal, low, moderate, high, or intense (Ginsberg *et al.* 2009). This represents an example of how the cloud infrastructure was coupled with big data and analytics to create something with relevance for population health.

In the future, other drivers to the use of the cloud will emerge. These include new generation sequencing techniques in health, which will provide potential applications in the domains of diagnostics for rare diseases, pharmacogenetics and related treatment guidance, cancer diagnostics and treatment guidance, microbiology, and predictive risk assessment. Transition from traditional methods (partial/targeted sequencing of particular genes) to full/whole-genome sequencing (FGS/WGS), also called high-throughput sequencing, is driving several changes related to data, including the generation of big data and its storage in the cloud. However, the potential of applying these sequencing techniques raises a number of questions such as, 'do we really want to know everything?' and, 'how do we know what to do?' Issues of data security and privacy, the legality of DNA registries, and the role of insurance companies also become paramount. Given the focus of genomic sequencing techniques on individuals from rich countries, its value for population-focused public health in the context of the resource-constrained environments of LMICs remains questionable.

Another trend in generating and storing big data in the cloud concerns the personal-based health record (PBHR), where health data related to the care of a patient is maintained by the patient. Many corporations such as Dossia, Microsoft Health Vault, and Google Health have taken up PBHR initiatives. Dossia promoted the slogan of 'Everyone has a unique health story; Dossia empowers you to author yours'. The Microsoft Health Vault, which urges people to 'take control of your own health', was started in 2007, but has been limited to the United States. It provides additional features for searching and accessing emergency health services, and a connection centre to enable direct upload to the PBHR, including from compatible devices for heart rate, blood pressure, and blood glucose. Google Health was another high-profile initiative which started in 2008, and soon shut down. People who had entered their personal data were told through the website that their data was lost forever. These different initiatives, which started about the same time, tell the same story: the potential of PBHRs is yet to be realized, and their collective impact is not yet evident. Such data and hosting infrastructure, again focused on individuals from rich countries, has limited relevance for public health in LMICs.

5.7.1 **Big data possibilities in low and middle-income countries**

Various LMICs are harnessing the potential of the cloud to shape big data initiatives. For example, India has come up with the National Health Portal to integrate all health-related data into a National Health Repository. The High Level Expert Group constituted by the Planning Commission for designing the scaling up of universal health coverage (UHC) (Planning Commission of India 2011) has made recommendations for developing a national health information technology network, which will be based on uniform standards to ensure interoperability deployed on the cloud. These initiatives, which largely represent policy statements, are fragmented, with a focus on establishing a technological infrastructure rather than supporting use to address significant public health challenges. Kenya is the first East African country to launch with World Bank funding an open data portal featuring information from government census, as well as economic, social, health, and education data. Users can potentially access information about healthcare facilities, doctors, and other information on their mobile phone with the use of the MedAfrica application (Germann *et al.* 2012). However, the challenge is of how the data will get continually updated and used meaningfully. Similar cloud and data initiatives are ongoing in Pakistan and Bangladesh.

In summary, the need for the cloud in LMICs is going to increase exponentially in the future, requiring simultaneous enhancement in capacities to manage and use data. These applications represent 'further from the machine applications' necessarily involving people, institutions, and a multiplicity of interests. These will raise various challenges, and also bring opportunities—these are discussed in the following section.

5.8 **Challenges and Opportunities for Health in Low and Middle-Income Countries**

5.8.1 **Key challenges**

Privacy and security

This represents key challenges with respect to the cloud and big data, particularly of reconciling potential benefits to public with risks to individual privacy (Appari and Johnson 2008). These are multifaceted challenges where technical developments continue to outpace legal advances, requiring interventions at multiple levels. For the individual, the question is how to ensure that informed consent is taken to enable personal data being placed in the cloud. There is fundamental ambiguity around the definition of personal data, and the rights associated with it. There are concerns about the anonymization of personal data, and often the technical solutions for de-identification are inadequate and vulnerable to hacker break-ins. At the organizational level, there are unknowns around contracts, for example, those between Ministries of Health and cloud service providers. Many ministries are bound by regulations that health data should not leave their national boundaries, and are not adequately informed on how to deal with the technical and institutional issues around the cloud.

Ownership

These concerns are significant for a variety of reasons given the multiplicity of actors involved, the geographical dispersion of where the cloud is, how data is used and reused, and the ambiguity of jurisdiction. Data is often collected by an agency for a particular purpose, and then further exploited by them and others for commercial purposes. For example, let us say that the Ministry of Health of a particular country is collecting name-based data on pregnant women in order to better monitor care. This data is stored in a national server, and is provided to an outsourcing agency to call the pregnant women to ascertain whether they have actually received the care that has been reported by the healthcare provider. Now there is the ownership question of whether the Ministry has the right to give personal data collected for a particular purpose to a third party, and what stops this party from using it for other purposes. They can further sell this data to firms dealing with, for example, baby products who will find value in this data for marketing. Similar ownership concerns of data are reflected in the ex UK Prime Minister David Cameron's statement: 'Every NHS patient would henceforth be a research patient whose medical record could be opened up for research by private healthcare research firms' (Tene and Polenesky 2013). This raises concerns of who does the research, on whom, and who benefits from its results. These asymmetries play out at individual, organizational, and national levels, especially from the perspective of LMICs. A key challenge here is to see how data on the cloud for public health can be positioned as a 'public good' to be used for the larger benefit of the population.

Epistemological dilemmas

These challenges relate to how knowledge is accessed. The traditional models of public health knowledge were based on a hypothetic-deductive logic followed by epidemiologists, involving the development of a priori hypothesis about a phenomenon (e.g. testing the correlation between smoking and cancer), establishing experiments or clinical trials based on scientifically defined criteria (of sample sizes, control groups, and statistical tests), and the execution of these experiments to develop 'a truth' about the phenomenon and make statistical generalizations with accompanying confidence levels. In contrast, big data analytics emphasizes identifying correlations retrospectively between different types of data often collected for other purposes. Without a guiding conceptual framework, finding such correlations using sophisticated data analytic techniques, backed with strong computing power may pick up many confounding incidental correlations with limited biological or social plausibility. Could this trend imply the 'death of theory' in favour of correlation-driven post-hoc analysis? A further implication concerns who drives this knowledge generation—will it be the epidemiologists with domain-specific knowledge, or will it be the cloud, IT, and big data specialists and corporations (like Google) who have the IT and big data analytics resources? If it is the latter, it will create natural power and knowledge asymmetries between the public health specialists and the big data and cloud specialists in the new economy. The cloud comes with the danger of creating complex analytical models and technological black boxes not accessible to public health practitioners. This puts at risk the concerns of patient safety and care.

Infrastructure

How the cloud infrastructures are designed, developed, evolved, and maintained are significant challenges for LMICs. The infrastructure required is necessarily complex, involving multiplicity of stakeholders, technological platforms, data types, and involves high financial investments. With respect to design, a key concern relates to enabling effective participation from patients and public health professionals, given the rising domination of the IT and data specialists, and resource-rich cloud providers causing dangers of vendor lock-ins and a threat to the sustainability of systems. There are extreme challenges of governance in forging sustainable partnerships and making choices in an environment where technologies are always evolving, new platforms are emerging, and existing ones becoming obsolete and unsupported, with high upgrade costs. This exacerbates the challenge of the already inherent power and knowledge asymmetries in the design and upkeep of such infrastructures.

Capacity strengthening

These challenges have historically plagued healthcare organizations in LMICs lacking the established technical capacities and cadres of specialists to even support reform efforts of their routine HMIS computerization. The use of the cloud raises the bar of capacity requirements significantly. Restrictions typically exist on new recruitments in public sector organizations, creating dependencies on external expertise and donor funds with obvious implications on sustainability and scalability. Under the framework of the cloud and big data, the demands on capacity, both in type and scale, will be far more acute than required for routine HMIS reform efforts. The use of cloud-based techniques requires a new breed of professionals who are IT savvy, understand systems and servers, and also have a good understanding of the domain to support analytical work. These capacities do not currently exist, and educational institutions are not incorporating these issues in their curriculum. The high cost of such skilled personnel, who are in high demand within the global marketplace, makes it difficult for health ministries in LMICs to compete for resources effectively.

In summary, effective leveraging of the potential for cloud infrastructure is fraught with major challenges, technological, data-related, institutional, and legal in nature, spanning levels of the individual, institutions, and the nation. Addressing them is a non-trivial task, which will take years and decades rather than months to implement. Furthermore, building appropriate capacity is a moving target, as the skill sets required are constantly changing. However, on the positive side, these challenges come along with some opportunities, and these are discussed in the next section.

5.8.2 Key opportunities

Supporting transitions in models of healthcare delivery

Cloud-supported data initiatives can potentially provide the impetus to support transitions from *disease to patient-based*; and, from *reactive to proactive* models of healthcare. While patient-based case sheets have always been available manually, IT can enable its systematic storage, rapid sharing, and longitudinal follow-up. Making these models operational assumes a high degree of reliance on access to cloud infrastructure, which is currently limited in LMICs. Many LMICs have constitutionally defined healthcare as a state (or district) rather than central/federal government subject, although in practice care is typically organized around donor-supported vertical national-level top-down disease-based models. While much success has been achieved with respect to the fight against polio, malaria, tuberculosis, and HIV, there are associated challenges of fragmentation and weak complementarity across programmes. In the UHC approach, a primary focus can be built on the patient, and the range of diseases s/he will experience during a lifetime. This requires data that is continuous, real time, covers the lifetime, and is pertaining to aspects in addition to healthcare, such as financial, social, lifestyle, and demographic-related. This requires the collection and processing of such different types of data on a continuous and long-term basis, and analytics of historical trends supported by cloud infrastructure. With improvements in software, techniques of aggregation moving from patient-based to aggregate data, and cloud hosting infrastructure, public health interventions can potentially be based on more accurate and relevant base data.

The transition from reactive to proactive models of healthcare will come with the shift from providing care to only those who *come to the health facility*, to entire populations in the service area. In a reactive model, many people and diseases remain invisible, thus not receiving the desired care. The example of diabetes is a classic case, where often a majority of the population remain oblivious to their diabetic condition or tendency, and reach the facility often in an advanced stage of the disease. Having a public health programme that provides annual check-ups and combining it with systems that record key health encounters and store all relevant historical data, available and accessible on the cloud, can potentially lead to early detection and management of the disease. Reorganizing healthcare delivery is, of course, primarily a matter of the health system, but IT can support this process in terms of managing databases, identifying who is being excluded, ensuring follow-up, measuring outcomes, and other such issues. Also, IT can allow data from different databases to be combined to make determinations that were previously not possible.

Addressing the challenge of scale

Scale refers to the ability of a system or an intervention to expand from the position it started from, across dimensions of geography, numbers, functionalities, use, vertically (across administrative levels), and horizontally (across business units, such as different health programmes at the district). Cloud-supported infrastructures can potentially enable health information systems to scale, and the internet and social media provide the possibility to collect data from widely distributed sources on an ongoing and real time basis, and of different granularities. Analyses and outputs from these applications can be disseminated to a larger audience and on a real time basis, and enables public involvement in implementing interventions. Cloud hosting of applications can allow for upgrades and support from technical teams located globally, and made available to health units distributed locally (e.g. all health facilities in a district), thus helping to surmount some capacity-related limitations. Improved sustainability will strengthen scaling when complemented with institutional measures of budgeting, and enabling regulation and partnerships between different stakeholders.

Ability to access low-cost and community-based software solutions

The growth of open source communities and crowd sourcing efforts towards building and maintaining data initiatives on the cloud implies that national governments and other information users can access more cost-effective technical solutions compared to those provided by proprietary vendors. An example is the University of Oslo's coordinated health information systems programme (HISP) network around the open source application DHIS 2, which is now in the process of being deployed (at different levels of maturity) in about 50-plus countries. The increasing maturing of open source health applications like DHIS 2 and OpenMRS means that countries can now access these products without having to reinvent the wheel, and thus receive financial investments directed primarily towards implementation and building capacity, rather than on developing software. The ability to draw upon community resources to respond to the changing needs of the health system allows for speedier response time without compromising quality.

Enabling more effective surveillance of diseases

Strengthening systems for mortality and morbidity reporting is a key challenge for national governments and global entities like the World Health Organization. The success of existing networks like INDEPTH and ALPHA, which have relied significantly on cloud infrastructure, has helped to strengthen mortality reporting systems by bringing together researchers from different countries to collect, analyse and disseminate data on a longitudinal basis, and conduct capacity building programmes regionally. The ALPHA network, which started in 2005, links existing African HIV cohort studies and runs training workshops to facilitate replication of analyses of demographic correlates and consequences of HIV infection. They undertake comparative studies and meta-analyses on comparable data sets, imposing common formats on data collection, storage, and analysis. Similarly, the INDEPTH network spans 20 countries in Africa, Asia, and Oceania, connecting researchers through a global network of health and demographic surveillance systems. The network has contributed to the development of data repositories, dissemination of analysed statistics, and organization of various capacity building programmes. While these networks are already taking advantage of cloud infrastructure and data analytic techniques, current technical advancements can help further strengthen these networks, and help create new ones.

5.9 Inductive Building of Design Principles: Use of the Cloud in Low and Middle-Income Countries

We now draw upon the guiding Expanded PHI approach to derive design principles for approaching the challenges and opportunities offered by the cloud and big data to LMICs. A guiding principle here is to view the cloud as being beyond a technical artefact and to ensure its use for strengthening population health.

5.9.1 **Enable a more sensitized engagement of development partners**

The scale of effort required to make the cloud and big data operational in LMICs will necessarily require the involvement of development partners and international institutions of public health. They play multiple roles—from funding technical support, global monitoring of diseases, dealing with health crises and emergencies such as Ebola, and advising national governments on strengthening data systems and supporting infrastructure. A focus of future efforts of development partners must be on supporting the creation of the cloud infrastructure, including its technical, institutional, and governance complexities. LMICs cannot address these issues on their own, given the technical complexities and financial investments required. To date, development partners have not provided adequate attention to cloud infrastructure, and this must necessarily become an important focus, including the building of public–private partnerships to enable development. As the role of external aid reduces, especially for emerging economies, the role that development partners play now, could and should shift to enable collaborations with international public health institutions and their national counterparts. The University of Oslo programme is one good example of such a shift taking place. In anticipation of these changes, public health organizations should start developing their capacities in these areas of knowledge generation and management —which are currently not included in their priorities list.

5.9.2 **Build mutual synergies between national health information systems and cloud initiatives**

There are various initiatives being undertaken by development partners, universities, and research groups on initiatives involving the cloud and big data, which are more often than not independent of national HIS strengthening efforts. A typical example of this is the US President's Emergency Plan For AIDS Relief (PEPFAR)'s global initiative of implementing their information systems across about 50 countries using a cloud-based infrastructure. PEPFAR is using the DHIS 2 platform, which is also used by the Ministries of Health in a majority of the targeted countries. While the ministries running these systems will typically be short on resources running their systems, the PEPFAR partners will be well resourced. The same holds for other development partners using the same DHIS 2 platform—they will all be better resourced than the ministries in a typical African country. For example in

Burundi, the Ministry of Health has been implementing the DHIS 2 platform for their routine health data, with limited funding and a shortage of human resources capacity. However, both the World Bank-funded RBF (result-based financing) programme and the PEPFAR are also implementing the DHIS 2 platform in Burundi and they have sufficient resources. The key question is therefore how synergies, especially institutional, can be established so as to support the Ministry of Health. During a discussion between the three parties on how synergies could be developed, shared training and support mechanisms were among the suggested modalities. However, nothing concrete has so far emerged. It is clear that the infrastructure, capacity, and network of support being developed for PEPFAR and other development partners and non-govermental organizations, such as in this example from Burundi, definitely could add synergy to the national HIS infrastructure, despite currently being separate. Policy guidelines are required to support the building of synergies, especially in gap areas in LMICs, such as in the monitoring of mortality and morbidity. Building such mutual synergies across systems and programmes requires the support of a cloud-enabled infrastructure which is proactively directed through policy and funding efforts within national priority frameworks.

5.9.3 Support the establishment of cloud and data science expertise in low and middle-income countries

Development partners and Ministries of Health should seek to establish expertise in the country for cloud infrastructure and big data analytic techniques. This requires sensitively designed initiatives to promote the development of hybrid skills in ICTs, cloud infrastructure and its governance, data analytics, systems integration, interpretation and use of data, and also health systems issues, such as those of regulation. National centres of excellence in health data science will help develop and propagate state of the art knowledge through workshops and short courses, forging partnerships with leading universities in order to build capacities at national and state levels. Such centres of expertise become centres of excellence only when they can grow beyond being satisfied in the role of conduits for dissemination of knowledge and skills to becoming partners in the active generation of knowledge and theorization.

5.9.4 Build regulatory frameworks to protect ethical and legal issues

Ministries need to provide leadership with the establishment of an enabling regulatory and governance environment to effectively address ethical, legal, and intellectual property-related issues at the multiple levels of the individual, health facility, Ministries of Health, and society. Issues to be addressed in these frameworks include: gaining consent prior to data collection; definition of personal data; anonymization of data; right to be forgotten; relevant jurisdiction; and liability related issues. Such a comprehensive regulatory environment will help to alleviate any mistrust that people may have about these new initiatives, and protect their rights in situations of conflict and disagreements. Useful learning for LMICs can come from the rich countries who have been grappling with these solutions for a longer time. For example, Norway has a system of disease registries supported through strong legislation. While LMICs will of course need to adapt such legislation to their respective contexts, a general learning to be gained is the fundamental need for such legislation to accompany the adoption of health data registries.

5.10 **References**

Appari, A. and Johnson, M.E. (2008). Information Security and Privacy in Healthcare: Current State of Research [Online]. Available at: http://www.ists.dartmouth.edu/library/416.pdf [Accessed: 24 October 2014].

Beardsley, S., Enriquez, L., Grijpink, F., Sandoval, S., Spittaels, S., and Strandell-Jansson, M. (2014). *Business Driven Technology*. McGraw Hill, New York, NY.

Germann, S., Jabry, A., Njogu, J., and Osumba R. (2012). The Illness of 'Pilotitis' in mHealth- Early Lessons from the KimMNCHip partnerships in Kenya. Global Health Forum [Online]. Available at: http://ghf.g2hp.net/2011/12/07/2154/#.VJARStKUeS8 [Accessed: 5 December 2014].

Ginsberg, J., Mohebbi, M.H., Patel, R.S., Brammer, L., Smolinski, M.S., and Brilliant, L. (2009). Detecting influenza epidemics using search engine query data. *Nature*, 457(7232), 1012–14.

Grossman, R.E. and Siegel , K.P. (2014). Organisational models for big data and analytics, *Journal of Organisational Design*, 3(1), 20–5.

Hoberg, P., Wallersheim, J., and Krcmar, H. (2012). The business perspective on cloud computing—A literature review of research on cloud computing. *AMCIS 2012 proceedings*.

Jolliffe, B., Poppe, O., Adaletey, D., and Braa, J. (2015). Models for online computing in developing countries: issues and deliberations. *Information Technology for Development*, 21(1), 151–61.

Laney, D. (2001). 3D data management. Controlling data volume, variety and veracity [Online]. Available at: https://blogs.gartner.com/doug-laney/files/2012/01/ad949-3D-Data-Management-Controlling-Data-Volume-Velocity-and-Variety.pdf Date: 6 February 2001. *Business Impact. File 949* [Accessed: 19 July 2016].

Mell, P., and Grance, T. (2011). The NIST Definition of Cloud Computing: Recommendations of Keen, J., Calinescu, R., Paige, R., and Rooksby, J. (2013). Big data + politics = open data. *Policy and Internet* the National Institute of Standards and Technology. NIST Special Publication 800-145 [Online]. Available at: http://csrc.nist.gov/publications/nistpubs/800-145/SP800-145.pdf [Accessed: 1 October 2015].

Normandeau, K. (2013). Beyond Volume, Variety and Velocity is the Issue of Big Data Veracity [Online]. Available at: http://insidebigdata.com/2013/09/12/beyond-volume-variety-velocity-issue-big-data-veracity [Last accessed: 1 July 2015].

Pentland A., Reid, T.G., and Heibeck T. (2013), Big Data and Health. Revolutionizing Medicine and Public Health, Report of the Big Data and Health, Working Group, WISH Big Data Health Report [Online]. Available at: http://www.wish-qatar.org/app/media/382 [Accessed: 22 November 2014].

Planning Commission of India (2011). High Level Expert Group Report on Universal Health Coverage for India. Constituted by Planning Commission of India, submitted before Parliament of India [Online]. Available at: http://planningcommission.nic.in/reports/genrep/rep_uhc0812.pdf [Last accessed 1 October 2015].

Purkayastha, P., Braa, J. (2013). Big data analytics for developing countries– using the cloud for operational BI in health. *Electronic Journal of IS in Developing Countries*, 59(6), 1–17.

Sahay, S., Nicholson, B., and Krishna, S. (2003). *Global IT Outsourcing: Software Development Across Borders*. Cambridge University Press, Cambridge, UK.

Silva, L.O. (2002). Outsourcing as an improvisation: A case study in Latin America. *The Information Society*, 18(2), 129–38.

Tene, O. and Polenetsky (2013). Big data for all: privacy and user control in the age of analytics. *Northwestern Journal of Technology and Intellectual Property*, 11(5), 240–72.

Vaughan-Nichols (2015). The public cloud is losing some of its luster [Online]. Available at: http://blogs.csc.com/2015/07/15/the-public-cloud-is-losing-some-of-its-luster/ [Last accessed: 1 October 2015].

Winner, L. (1978). *Autonomous technology: technics-out-of-control as a theme in political thought*. Mit Press, Cambridge, MA.

Zuboff, S (2014) A Digital Declaration: Speech. [Online]. Available at: http://www.faz.net/aktuell/feuilleton/debatten/the-digital-debate/shoshan-zuboff-on-big-data-as-surveillance-capitalism-13152525.html [Last accessed: 1 October 2015].

Chapter 6

Institutions as Barriers and Facilitators of Health Information Systems Reform

6.1 The Need to Describe the Institutional Perspective

In Chapters 1 and 2, we defined the key differences between health IT and health informatics, such that the latter term includes the institutional context wherein information technology is embedded—and this includes the way in which information is produced, distributed, and used. We further defined public health informatics as the subdiscipline of health informatics which concerns the health of populations. Finally, we introduced the term Expanded Public Health Informatics (PHI) to denote that the informatics of populations is not distinct from healthcare informatics, which focuses on the healthcare of individuals but is increasingly built upon and subsumes the latter into itself. Thus, healthcare informatics becomes a subset of Expanded PHI.

We turn our attention now, in this chapter, to explaining what we mean by institutions, and how different theories of institutions can help to better analyse the challenges of public health informatics. Institutional theory has been used widely in information systems and organizational studies to understand different kinds of organization settings, and the challenges faced in different kinds of change efforts. In recent years, this theory has been increasingly used to study the role of health information systems (HIS) within the context of public sector organizations in low and middle-income countries (LMICs). While in general, institutional theory has been criticized for focusing more on explaining stability rather than change, new strands of institutional theory provide a rich repertoire of concepts such as contradictions, logics, deinstitutionalization, institutional entrepreneurship, and a greater focus on human agency and cognitive structures that help understand change. While this field of study is very vast, spanning more than five decades of scholarship, in this chapter we focus on describing an institutional perspective, which helps to understand the role of HIS within an Expanded PHI framework.

6.2 **Building an Institutional Perspective to Understand Expanded PHI**

We attempt to develop an institutional perspective by approaching Expanded PHI at two levels—the macro and the micro, and their inter-connections. First, we provide a brief introduction to the institutional perspective.

6.2.1 **An introduction to the institutional perspective**

Fogel and North (1993) in their Nobel prize acceptance speech state, 'If institutions are the rules of the game, organizations and their entreprenurs are the players.'

Thus, a district health system—a legally defined entity—can be seen in this definition as an organization referring to the persons who are working on the team for a common set of objectives; or as an institution, as defined by the different rules which govern its mandate and functioning. Within the public health settings, we can conceptualize the medical profession, the district and state health systems, or the local governments, and other enforcement agencies as institutions with their respective formal and informal rules.

North emphasizes that the rules that define institutions can be both formal and informal. While formal rules can be, for example, the Articles of Association defining the society, its human resource policy, informal rules represent the norms of behaviour, work culture, and unwritten conventions and traditions that often serve as facilitators or constraints to implementing change (North 1990). From a study of implementing the new monitoring and evaluation system in Mozambique, Piotti *et al.* (2006) observe that the more the overlap between the formal and informal, the greater is the chance for reform efforts to succeed. The reason for this is that formal mandates for change actively take into account the existing work systems. However, the danger here is that this may support continuation of the status quo, and thus little change may come about.

Institutions have been popularly described as socially constructed systems of rules, norms, and meanings under which social actors generate regularities of behaviour. This perspective helps to explain how the power of institutions can influence the adoption and institutionalization of new IT systems and practices in both developed and developing countries. Institutional pressures, such as the values and meanings underpinning an IT innovation, can influence its adoption and implementation contributing to organizational change (or not). Introduction of new HIS always involves tensions between existing institutional structures that promote stability and institutional features that encourage change, such as new Information and Communications Technologies (ICTs), and imperatives of modernity coming through different sources such as donor funding. Understanding the processes of technology-enabled change and health outcomes requires a more attentive analysis of the motives and actions of key social and political actors, and how these are embedded in a framework of formal rules and norms of behaviour. An example concerns the processes and structures in place to enable participation of health staff in technology design and development processes (Braa and Sahay 2012). These considerations point to the need for perspectives that provides a balanced account of the relationship between institutions, technology, and human agencies, representing the intention and capacity of individuals and organizations to engage with change.

6.2.2 **From a macro-institutional perspective**

Neo-classical economists generally perceive institutions as interference to the market system, which is considered to be the favoured mechanism for the allocation of resources. While traditionally health, education, and law enforcement were once viewed to be independent of the market system, today this is not the case as we see, for example, in the infiltration of private insurance and technology providers in all areas of healthcare including the public health domain. In a market-based framework of understanding, with an increase in market demand for information, suppliers of information would emerge and cater to this demand. The more efficient suppliers of information (who would implicitly deploy technology more effectively) would be rewarded with greater market presence. Optimal allocation of resources, even in the public health sector, is slowly being conceptualized as happenning under the aegis of the market. However, in the past few decades there has been increasing recognition of situations where market failure occurs due to information asymmetry, or due to moral hazards, or inherent in the nature of public goods. Many of these scenarios of market failure are widely acknowledged in the health sector, and this has had implications on public health informatics.

The recognition of market failure has led to a revival of interest in the role institutions play in ensuring optimal allocation of resources, leading to the rise of what has been termed 'new institutional economics'. Douglas North, Elinor Ostrom, and many other scholars have tried to analyse and theorize the different contexts and understandings of institutions, and how and where they function (or fail to function), and created the 'Institutional Analysis and Development (IAD) framework' to study these (Ostrom 2011). It informs us that institutions must be configured in certain ways—where consumer choice is still exercised and is transferred to institutional choice through the government or collectives/organizations. These theories call for different forms of institutional choice, thus enabling better allocations on the market. Institutions can overcome the causes of market failures, for example, by purchasing on behalf of individuals, and if people are allowed to make a choice, the institutions could mediate on their behalf.

However in most contexts of public health, peoples' ability to influence decisions with regard to healthcare priorities or the shape of heathcare institutions is limited. While IAD is useful to understand institutional influences in many contexts, it does not sufficiently explain how institutional choice occurs in situations characterized by asymmetry of information and a very unequal distribution of power. It does not help us predict how introduction of technology would be received in different scenarios or contexts. Just because a particular HIS has worked in one context, it does not mean it would work in another. And we need to look at other institutional theories that would help understand this. Earlier institutional perspectives looked at rules in relation to power. Weber's work on bureaucracy (Weber 1946), for example, defines the roles played by different elements in bureaucracy and types of authority that needed to be mobilized for institutions to be effective. This was criticized, as it was based on a premise that ideally all authorities act in the best interests in a disinterested way, although in real life it is never the case.

The principal–agent theory, also known as theory of agency, provides useful insights into understanding the role of institutions, especially in the presence of differing interests. The agent in this theory is one who makes decisions on behalf of, or that affect, another person or organization—the latter being called the 'principal'. Although it is expected that the agent would act on behalf of the principal, in practice his/her own interests and those of other principals would influence—and sometimes dominate—the decision-making process, a distortion magnified in cases of information asymmetry, when the principal does not have the knowledge required to know whether the agent is acting on his or her behalf or not.

In a purely market-based approach, the way forward is to provide appropriate incentives for agents to act in the way principals wish. In terms of game theory, this involves changing the rules of the game so that the self-interested rational choices of the agent coincide with the objectives of the principal. Therefore, attention shifts to building more and more innovative mechanisms of contracting and its supervision to ensure this 'harmony'. In a Weberian analysis, when faced with principal to agent misalignment, it would be the use of authority that would ensure the realignment.

In theories of political economy, the value of information and thereby its allocation is seen not as something set merely by supply and demand, but largely determined by the terms in which information is produced, distributed, and consumed. In most theories of political economy, institutions are seen as embedded in power relationships. Thus, an agent could have many principals—and which influence finally shapes the action of the agent, and to what degree, depends upon the balance of power between the principals and the agent itself. Changing the rules redefines the balance of powers, but so does the introduction of technology.

6.2.3 **A micro-level institutional perspective**

An interesting micro-level institutional perspective to understand the dynamics around HIS-enabled change is that of institutional work, which emphasizes a more agency-focused approach and its relation with technology. Various streams of work in institutional theory become relevant in building this perspective. One concerns the notion of the organizational field and the different actors which form the sphere of influence on work. For example, HIS introduction is shaped by the influences of ministries, donors, software vendors, and infrastructure providers. Together these entities and their influences form the organizational field. Often these influences are conflicting, and create contradictions which also carry with them the potential for change. For example, the varying influences of a donor promoting an open source-based HIS and the ministry favouring the proprietary system create a contradiction; and in resolving this, there is the inherent potential for change.

Another useful concept concerns institutional entrepreneurship which focuses on the role of particular actors in creating networks to disrupt existing power balances in the process of introducing change. These actors often have to deal with the paradox of trying to change institutions which they themselves are products of, and which by definition favour stability. The institutional entrepreneur would need to mobilize external resources and legitimacy to try and upset the existing power balance, and in this process move from the periphery to the core. This may be done to further the commercial interests of the entrepreneur, or it could be done to ensure that the changes being introduced are sustained and lead to the improvements in health sector performance. One example of a positive institutional entrepreneur role is the use that many national ministries have made of the Health Information Systems Programme (HISP) network, and the legitimacy that DHIS 2 has acquired to catalyse much-needed health sector reforms that lead to better information use and increased decentralization.

A supporting concept to institutional entrepreneurship is that of deinstitutionalization, which examines how existing institutions lose their legitimacy and get eroded, giving the space for new institutions to emerge and for a process of re-institutionalization to take place. Disruptive institutional work *cannot rest on mere efficiency arguments*, but involves the much harder task of dismantling sanctions, moral foundations, and beliefs supporting taken-for-granted behaviours and IT systems. Such work may trigger the reaction of political opponents who engage in 'defensive institutional work' to try and maintain existing practices which give them the power and legitimacy to continue. ICTs also carry with them particular institutional norms and values, and also different affordances—representing how individuals see these technologies to support their goal-oriented actions. Because these perceptions are shaped by the institutions under which the actors operate, the technologies themselves become institutionally shaped.

One way forward is to look at technology introduction as a process of negotiation. Or if we understand every institutional design to already be a result of past negotiations, then the process can be seen as technology introduction and re-negotiation. This then recognizes the need to follow the rules of negotiation, and accept the limits of negotiated solutions to enable progress. And we have to remind ourselves that however powerful the leadership, since the relationships of power are embedded in the design of institutions, no single person wherever situated would have such ability as to override all other sources of power. But as a corollary, without informed leadership it would not be possible to establish a negotiation or ensure the direction of change resulting from a negotiation.

In summary, a macro-institutional perspective based on principal–agent theories and political economy provides us a framework to understand, for example, the questions of technological choice. This, when complemented with a micro-perspective of institutional work, helps provide a lens to study the practice-level dynamics around technology introduction and use. Together they lead to a more holistic perspective of the role of institutions in shaping HIS reform processes.

6.3 Institutions in Which Health Information Systems Are Embedded

There are many institutions that come into play in the production, flow, and use of health information—represented as the information value chain. For simplicity we categorize them into the following broad categories.

i) The logic of healthcare institutions
ii) The logic of healthcare information management institutions
iii) The logic of public health decision-making institutions
iv) The logic of donor-funding institutions

These are now discussed.

6.3.1 The logic of healthcare institutions

These institutions are defined as those where healthcare providers perform their duties, which includes not only the provision of healthcare, but in the process as a corollary, the production of vast amounts of information. A doctor in a primary healthcare facility or a nurse providing outreach care can be seen as agents with multiple principals. First, the doctor acts on behalf of patients, making decisions around what medicines to give, and what diagnostics and referrals are required. Here information is required to enable quality and continuity of care. While today an electronic medical record is used to store and retrieve this data, previously it was done through manual case-sheets, nursing notes, prescriptions, and discharge summaries.

The doctor also acts on behalf of the employer, which is typically the Department of Health. In this case, in addition to the patient record, he/she is expected to maintain a record of services delivered which would justify and make accountable the consumables and other resources consumed. Further, there is the need to provide a periodic report of work done for purposes of monitoring and accountability, and also to inform on the health status of the population covered. In a hospital, a set of reports may be required for the hospital administration, another for the insurance agency for purposes of reimbursement, and various others for different health programmes like TB, Malaria, HIV, and so on. Typically each principal would push for the primacy of their own information needs, often without aligning with needs of other principals.

In this form of principal–agent relationship, the nurse or doctor may need to maintain over 20 records to support the multiplicity of principals to whom they must report. Repeated efforts to harmonize the needs of the different principals tend to fail, often leading to the development of informal institutions where the field nurse may draw columns in an existing register to record data which was otherwise not included. These informal inclusions tend to serve as constraints to new computerization efforts, as these workarounds tend to be invisible to the design process. The health worker would need to sit with these multiple registers once every month and cull out the aggregate numbers needed for the multiple reporting formats that she has to submit. This process of aggregation from these multiple registers containing her workarounds is a cumbersome process, understood only by the particular health worker, and subject to various calculation errors, compounded by the degree of disaggregation required. Computerization of such processes which are person-dependent and subjective is a complex process and prone to failure.

Sensitively and well-designed ICT systems can play an important role in streamlining these recording and reporting processes. The nurse or doctor could enter each health activity or event as a single line, based on the formal institution or rule that any one data element would be entered only once and by only one person. Electronically all information needed for providing follow-up care and referrals gets generated from this. The facility's monthly aggregate reports specific to different programmes can also be generated electronically by aggregating all the different patient-specific records. This enables reducing the burden of work for the data collector, and enables the provider to not only access individual records for follow-up, but also the aggregated reports useful in developing a better understanding of the local public health. Institutionally, for such a system to work, all principals—patient, individual programme managers, health facility manager, public health managers—have to align their needs with each other and communicate these to the provider, and each must respect the needs and responsibilities of the other. This is both an institutional and a technical requirement for alignment. The technical requirement for alignment can be missed, since often the design of the system is only aligned with the wants (as different from needs) of the top public health manager—whose grasp of the needs of all those down the value chain is very limited.

In practice, therefore, this alignment is seldom achieved, and the technology tends to become an additional burden of work on the service providers. Without the required alignment, the provider has to enter the same data into multiple systems and generate various reports for different principals. In addition, it does not make any existing work easier as it does not enable value-added functions like local analysis of data, or better quality of follow-up in patient care. The existing manual system is retained until such time as confidence is built in the new system, a stage which most often is never reached, thus causing parallel systems to continue.

New ICTs are seen as placing the health worker under a system of surveillance to strengthen work discipline, which creates an atmosphere of mistrust. This is natural for any bureaucracy—as the arm of state power—but stronger when inherited from colonial administration, where there was a deep suspicion of the population and the native workers. As some said in jest: 'the British invented the bureaucracy, and the Indians perfected it'. Sometimes this leads to resistance, when there is failure to comply with the institutional directions from the top. Resistance is heightened by the doctor as a professional. The medical profession as an institution privileges the doctor to make decisions and act in the best interests of the patients. This creates an information asymmetry, since the medical professional is accountable only to itself and to a notional professional supervision. Such a professional finds it almost a duty to *not* adhere to any non-professional institution for his/her individual behaviour. Nurses and pharmacists are also professionalized, but less privileged.

Some of these institutional tensions are highlighted through Case Study 6.1.

Case Study 6.1 mHealth Comes to Punjab

By 2010, Punjab, a state in North India, was doing relatively well with respect to their routine HMIS, using the DHIS 2 as their state data warehouse, while dealing with the usual problems of poor data quality, limited data use, and lack of feedback. A proof of concept for a mHealth pilot was done in 2009 by HISP India and NHSRC on the request of the Ministry of Health. The pilot aimed to establish the technical feasibility of a workflow where the field nurse would enter the monthly facility data into the java application on her mobile, and send the same by SMS to a central database. There was also potential for data to be analysed and then feedback sent to her mobile, so that work could be expedited. The pilot showed immense potential to improve timeliness of reporting, lessen the travel burden, and also possibly improve data quality. Feedback received directly on the phone could potentially trigger local action. It looked like a win-win situation for all.

The state government saw the possibilities from this pilot and decided to go to scale and take this across the state. No sooner had the mobiles been purchased and the implementation begun, than the key administrator behind the project changed. The new administrator, enthused by the possibilities of monitoring every worker, decided to distribute one phone per nurse, rather than one per facility. When there were sometimes two health workers in a facility, their work roles varied, and they could not really use the same data entry screens for reporting. To strengthen monitoring, the administrator introduced the institution of daily reporting of 12 data elements—which now could not be cast into indicators, since the denominators would differ for each. As a consequence, the data no longer contributed to the monthly HMIS report, which continued the old way—manually recorded on paper, brought to district headquarters, and entered in the system. A monitoring cell was also set up under the administrator at state headquarters to receive the reports, and then identify the errant field worker and act on that information.

The consequences of these changes could have been predicted. The introduction of the mobile increased the burden of work considerably and brought no visible benefits to the provider, made no improvement to data quality or use, and increased the atmosphere of mistrust. The existing chain of command where the field worker reported to the facility medical officer was short-circuited as the data went directly to the state server, leading to decreased accountability on this chain. But without the context of the field worker's everyday work, the reports could not be interpreted, making centralized monitoring completely ineffective. Resistance from the health staff increased, and they went on strike for nearly a month, protesting against this system of surveillance. The strike was successful in shifting daily monitoring to weekly, reducing the sense of ongoing surveillance. However, it continued as a redundant and parallel function.

An institutional interpretation of this case makes us aware of multiple factors, one being the administrator who focused on the daily report he wanted, ignoring the needs of other principals, and the need to coordinate and harmonize the multiple information needs into the design.

This takes us further into the institutional analysis, where it is seen that much of health sector reform involves shifting executive power from technical to general administrators, who are generally not equipped to understand the technical dimensions of public health, and instead focus only on the monitoring and controlling aspects. But more importantly, when they assume executive functions, they vacate their primary role of an institution builder, which involves creating rules and norms to enable alignment of the interests of different principals. The technical staff, being professionals, resist being placed in a subordinate relationship to the general administrator, and see it as a failure of the reform process; their own lack of knowledge about institutional design and how it impacts management does not help either. Unfortunately, even the general administrators find the unravelling of the grand vision of monitoring to be flawed, as discipline has such a limited role in managing of any workforce—especially a salaried organized workforce.

6.3.2 The logic of healthcare information management

Healthcare information management institutions are concerned with information systems management and the establishment, the function and evaluation of system design, and typically represent the components of the information systems lifecycle. Typically, this starts from expressing requirements, procuring a service provider to build the system, heightening of expectations of how digitization will solve a multitude of problems, and then a period of implementation, a readjustment of expectations, growing frustration and criticisms and mutual recrimination, leading to abandonment or obsolescence of the system, and its replacement through the next cycle. While such a cycle characterizes individual stand-alone systems serving a specific set of functions, there are other problems at the architectural level, such as those related to integration for both technical and institutional reasons. Architecture decisions are shaped by technology, markets, and increasingly the modern day institutions of e-governance. Institutions of governance, which we deal with in Chapter 9, are different from those of information management, which are concerned more with operational decisions such as who sources information, channels it, processes it, and provides it to users who are distinct from them. We present Case Study 6.2 from Tajikistan to understand the key institutions that were influencing the health management information systems (HMIS) reform process in the country.

6.3.3 **The institution of procurement: A key constraint to health management information systems reform**

Key institutions that define HIS management are those concerned with the procurement and managing of IT services, and the IT service providers themselves. The rules that govern procurement and the organization that administers these rules tend to be extremely rigid with little scope for innovation. One set of problems relates to the fact that most rules have been developed for procurements where specifications are clear and it is relatively easier to ascertain delivery and make payments. Procurement of services is more complex, but essentially the principles in use are similar to those in use for any commodity. The bid is broken up into a technical and a financial part—and only those who qualify on the technical bid are considered for the financial bid. It is expected that if the technical capacity required is clearly and competently stated, low quality, and non-serious bids can always be eliminated. These tenders place certain entry barriers—like having done similar work before or having a minimum company size and revenue, ostensibly to eliminate low quality bids. Often these thresholds are so high that all but two or three large companies get eliminated. In particular, low budget resourceful open source-based firms and NGOs get excluded even from participation in such tenders, even though they may provide good quality technical solutions.

Procurement gives great importance to process and a very strict and literal adherence to rules. Two completely contradictory factors work to shape this. One is the fear that officers involved in making decisions are accused of being corrupt. The second is that there are various firms who are willing to pay bribes to secure contracts. The process is so rule-dense that it is easy to hold up files for one reason or another and without un-billed payments the files just do not move at all. But also necessarily some rules have to be overridden and few will take the risk without a monetary consideration. This also works to the advantage of the corporate healthcare IT vendor and against the small scale

(continued on page 140)

Case Study 6.2 Institutional Influences on HMIS Reform Process in Tajikistan

This case study (Sahay *et al.* 2010) examines the key institutions that challenge the introduction of ICT-based HMIS reforms in the context of a post-Soviet economy—Tajikistan.

Tajikistan is unique in many respects. It is a Central Asian country about which little, if anything, has been published in the mainstream information systems and development literature. Gaining independence after the downfall of the Soviet Union in 1991, Tajikistan experienced an extremely rocky period, with a prolonged civil war and the loss of the supporting Soviet financial and social infrastructure. The country experiences an extreme climate, has a long and porous border with the war-ravaged Afghanistan, and has suffered a food and energy crisis of huge proportions. It has also seen the exodus of many trained people due to weak employment and decreasing social opportunities at home. Tajikistan faces urgent public health problems. The demise of the Soviet economic base, followed by civil war, has led to a surge in various communicable diseases in the last two decades, and this coupled with poor nutrition and polluted water has contributed to a drop in life expectancy among the population.

Acknowledging the key role that ICTs can play in development and public health management, the Asian Development Bank established the Health Sector Reform Project in 2005, with the aim of creating various reform initiatives, including those relating to HMIS. The reform process has been ongoing over the last decade, and has involved various donors and consultants, each focusing on particular aspects of HMIS reform including the definition of indicators, the redesign of the paper-based systems, the selection of software, customization, and pilot testing. This process of reform has been long and arduous, primarily because of the challenges related to countering the policies of the existing institutions left behind by the Soviet legacy, which favoured a large manual system based on a centralized planning model.

In the initial study of the existing situation of the HMIS in 2007, two dominant institutional logics were identified. The first related to central control of the HMIS under the medical statistics division (MedStat), which saw HMIS as the tool for generating annual statistics for their different principals, including the Parliament, the President's Office, and the donor community. The central control of the statistics wing was a legacy from the Soviet rule that mandated the collection of large amounts of data and sending to the national level for making prospective five-year plans. The concept of data collection for supporting local-level action or providing feedback to lower levels was largely absent.

The software used for generating these statistics was based on the out-of-date FoxPro platform, where data was entered on 37 reporting forms and generated for different categories of organization units, mostly on an annual basis. The software was not capable of generating any indicators (such as percentages or rates per thousand that required calculation with a numerator and denominator). Neither was the software capable of generating graphs and charts, and only statistical tables could be created. To develop graphical outputs, the statistics generated were manually fed into a separate programme, where indicators were generated, and manually uploaded into a national website.

The other dominant institutional influences came from the primacy of paper-based systems. These paper systems tried to include, at an extraordinary level of detail, all kinds of data which were also products of the Soviet legacy. For example, a data element still being collected in the routine HMIS was 'airplane vibrations heard', obviously an obscure legacy of the war times. There was a multiplicity of programmes, some electronic and some based on paper, but none could electronically speak to any other, despite all being under the control of the National Statistics division (called MedStat). Below the level of the 37 forms that corresponded to the different health programmes (with a great deal of overlap and redundancies) were another 367 recording forms used at the primary health facilities to record the provision of basic services. The reporting forms were poorly designed and comprised multiple subforms. For example, the form titled 'Treatment Prophylactic Activity of Facility' contained about 50 subforms, covering 1836 data elements and spanning 75 pages.

Given the huge amount of the data to be reported (about 30,000 data elements) on a routine basis, the extremely weak HMIS-related resources, and the view that reporting was an irrelevant exercise, data quality and use of information obviously suffered. These massive reams of paper could not provide the doctors with the data they immediately needed, which led to various local improvizations. For example, the Infectious Diseases Department at a central district created an 'emergency form' that listed eight essential diseases and this was used for local action.

Efforts to rationalize and computerize had to confront both these institutional legacies of central control and dominance of paper. The forms had multiple columns against a particular data element; for example the

'Immunization' section would have multiple age categories associated with it, and also a column for 'totals'. Although officials were told that they did not need to manually enter the 'total' since the computer would automatically generate it, they continued to replicate the paper forms to the last detail. Similarly, there were logos on the paper which could not be modified at all in terms of placement, even though the reporting forms could be made to look more elegant with minor changes.

Computerization efforts thus struggled with dismantling the existing institutions and replacing them with new. It is only now, about seven to eight years after the reform process started that the systems have been redesigned, and the open source DHIS 2 has been used to deploy the revised systems at a national scale. However, creating institutions of local use of information will take many more years.

Source: data from Sahay S, Sæbø JI, Mekonnen SM, and Gizaw, AA. Interplay of institutional logics and implications for deinstitutionalization: case study of HMIS implementation in Tajikistan. *Information Technologies and International Development*, Volume 6, Issue 3, pp. 19, Copyright © 2010 USC Annenberg School for Communication and Journalism.

service provider, who either does not have the resources or is often ideologically against bribes.

Procurement of ICT services for healthcare is challenging because of the difficulties in spelling out its requirements, which are extremely dynamic and keep changing, even as systems are being deployed. In addition, firms with high turnovers who get the contracts for public health work do not send their 'A teams' for implementation, because the volume of revenues is relatively small. Maintenance support and its cost are also difficult to estimate, and change management efforts are not easily quantifiable. Finally, as users become familiar, more users join and more needs arise, necessitating changes in software. Proprietary vendors tend to withdraw once their payment is made, and will wait for a new contract before responding to these necessary changes. A situation arises where the user is locked-in with a single vendor, and is forced to continue even with declining service quality.

There are also institutional challenges within the service provider. Most IT firms have limited public health skills, and work with the assumption that the customer can specify their needs accurately. In practice this does not happen. Often, because of the multiplicity of principals involved, the provider tends to be obliged to listen to the top player, even though he may not be primary for the design of the system. Usually the top player, the Secretary of Health, has a presumption of the information needs which are at variance with the ground realities. It is not common for this top player to be specifying requirements such as the need for automated correlations of deaths and causes, while the reality on the ground is for strengthening data management processes. This problem is exacerbated where the top player is a general civil servant—a bird of passage—who will move from the top position before any ICT project can become sustainable. The Punjab mHealth case demonstrates this transience which has adverse effects on the projects.

There are small start-up firms and niche firms which could take on a task that requires long-term maintenance, such as building and maintaining websites. But such firms would not meet the pre-qualification criteria set for the larger tenders. Very often, the complexities of procurement and the interests of donors add layers between the service provider and the user. In the almost inevitable stage of criticism and mutual recrimination, the service providers find it easier to tell the donor, who is the paymaster, that the problems of implementation lie in the national public health institutions, and deflect any criticisms from themselves.

Products based on open standards and open source principles where the source code is mandatorily made available lend themselves to evolution within the public health context. But large firms are less open to open source, as policy and their brand influence is such that their views prevail. Eligibility criteria for participation in bids are tweaked so as to remove many open source players, even though they are financially better placed, and also have ethical arguments associated with their bids.

Finally, this whole process of selection and retention is based on competition—both for getting the best price and the best product. However where there is so much uncertainty and change—reflected in the inability to freeze requirements—and with so much work required in capacity building, hand-holding, troubleshooting, and when products themselves have to be very dynamic, it raises the need for models that promote collaboration. A community of practice, where different IT firms working on different products could actually talk to each other and learn from each other could be very productive, but in an environment based on competition, and pregnant with information asymmetries, this is extremely difficult to achieve. The way forward rests on innovation at both ends—changing the rules of procurement of IT firms so they are better suited to the needs of the public health system, and changing the nature of the firm itself. Many funding agencies are beginning to see the logic of this, but for national governments, the task of bringing in these changes is much more complex.

6.3.4 **The logic of public health decision-making institutions**

First—who are the institutional entities that serve as custodians of information?

The single most important user of public health information is the public health leadership of the government—as present in the Ministry of Health. In nations with a federal structure, the Ministries of Health at both the centre and the state (or province) matter. The greater the decentralization of powers to provinces and to districts, the greater the role of users at those levels, which eventually become more important than the central structure. Government decision-making institutions are not monoliths—there is a bewildering and exasperating complexity within—where it becomes difficult to even figure out who makes the decisions. This is especially true for robust and noisy democracies like India. Often, the rule of making a decision is *not* making one, but postponing it into an indeterminate future. Even more difficult to fathom is what role information plays, if at all, in decision-making. Fortunately however, we can make a much clearer statement of how information is processed and presented to the decision makers. We can also from our case studies examine how different decision makers influence the content and even the form of the health information flow. In every setting, an individual as an institutional entity serves as the custodian of information.

Who that source of power is represents a historical legacy, described in institutional theory as path dependence, a classical problem of institutional capacity and management. The historical process by which an organization evolves, and the distribution of powers within and the politics without, are greater determinants of the path taken than the technical merit or responsiveness to the needs. Not that these do not change—they do—but slowly and partially, and often involving many costly hit-and-miss efforts. A classical problem here is how ministries still continue to focus on raw numbers and not indicators, and this, despite a decade of learning, has been difficult to change.

Every health ministry has some set of functionaries or a division, which either by design or through practice becomes responsible for collecting information from different sources and providing it to policy makers and to the public. In many nations, this function is allocated to the statistics division within the Ministry of Health, comprising of a group of statisticians. In some countries, it is the planning cell, and increasingly, we see the role of the IT group becoming more powerful, given the heightened role of technology.

The statistics cadre is an interesting feature of most governments—particularly those with a colonial past. The staff typically comprises qualified postgraduates or doctorates in statistics, who do not belong to one particular department, and could in rotation be placed in any ministry (such as education, health, child welfare, or agriculture) in the centre or the state. They tend to enjoy, both by the knowledge they deal with and also formal administrative relationships, a degree of autonomy from the department (such as Health) they are attached to. The colonial legacy has defined their roles as custodians, collecting information from different sources, compiling it, and presenting it to the decision makers, such as the Secretary of Health, the Planning Commission, Department of Statistics, and sometimes even to the offices of the Prime Minister and the President.

The strength of the statisticians is in designing population-based surveys, especially the sampling strategy and data analysis. The relative autonomy they enjoy empowers them to present their reports, even if it was bad news. But there is also considerable incentive to give good news and downplay the bad, as these reports find their way to the Parliament, Planning Commission, Finance Ministry, Auditor General's office, and other relevant bodies. It thus becomes essential for the statisticians to present the Ministry's performance in a good light, and this involves a struggle to balance contradictory needs—of sharing facts to facilitate planning, while ensuring the reports look good. Giving the 'final' verdict on the data thus becomes the privilege of the statisticians.

With the increasing proliferation of IT, the game may be changing, with IT departments (and vendors) becoming important spheres of influence. Different configurations tend to emerge with alliances being created between IT and statistics, sometimes one taking a more powerful role than the other. The statisticians tend to be usually quite clueless about the developments in ICTs and fall easy prey to the dazzling marketing pitch of IT firms. By definition, they also have only a minimal understanding of public health and are dependent on programme managers and donors to define the data sets and analysis needs. A key focus area for them is data quality, where their statistical knowledge lends itself to the analysis of data trends and outliers, but often all with raw numbers and not as indicators which are difficult to generate because of the perennial problem of denominators. What seems to be emerging in many nations are central-level alliances of statisticians, IT technicians, and programme managers to map requirements, largely ignoring the information needs of the district and mid-level managers and service providers below. Studying the lock-ins to particular technologies and vendors is often crucial in defining the nature of the problem.

At the level of the hospital, the custodian is usually the doctor, who brings a different perspective (and set of problems) compared to statisticians. In hospitals, the problem of information often is reduced to 'Oh, doctors!' While no doubt, there is considerable resistance that arises from professional perceptions and privilege, an institutional work perspective warrants a closer look at the rules governing the work of doctors. A hospital information system needs to allow the doctor some flexibility in what data is to be recorded for an individual, and with what level of certainty this is expressed. The doctor needs to have a space to indicate the level of uncertainty between the diagnosis and treatment plan in the communication made with the patient. Often doctors provide treatment on purely presumptive and even speculative grounds—a necessary exercise of clinical judgement. But most hospital information systems demand that every patient must have a precise diagnosis which corresponds to one unique standard treatment that every doctor will know and follow. In many settings, doctors reject this need for compliance to certainty, and tend to resist the introduction of the hospital information system. Without the doctors' support, the system cannot become effective, and the doctors continue as the custodians of clinical information, which cannot be made visible to the levels above.

In summary, the question of who are the institutional custodians of information is an important one for the Ministry of Health, while analysing the value and role of information. Custodians will vary with the levels of administration of the organization and the nature of work they do. In countries with strong colonial legacies and in nations with Soviet-style centralized planning traditions, primacy is usually to the statisticians, who in the contemporary context of change need to make alliances with IT teams and programme managers in order to maintain their role as custodians. In hospital facilities, the doctors often serve as the custodians, often to continue the primacy of norms coming from the medical profession that are aligned to the need for coping with the uncertainty between diagnosis, treatment, and patient communication. The combination of the macro- and micro-perspectives of institutions helps to understand how and in what form information becomes available for processing.

Second—what institutional processes link information and decision-making?

The custodians of information shape what information, in what form and tone of expression (good or bad news), gets presented, and to whom. This leads us to the question: does neither planning nor resource allocation become information driven?

As discussed in Chapter 3, most planning and policy decisions often happen by political processes involving considerable negotiations among key stakeholders, with information playing only a limited role. Public choice theories are relevant to our analysis, to examine how policy decisions are made, and who are the drivers of decision-making. A key driver in public health tends to be collection of information for satisfying the monitoring and accountability functions. The Central Ministry of Health is accountable to Parliament, Prime Minister, Planning Commission, Finance Ministry, Auditor General, often to courts of law, and increasingly to media and civil society. Similarly, the state or province and district levels have their own accountability mechanisms which shape what information is collected (or not), and its flow, use, and content.

In India, during the first five years of the National Rural Health Mission reform process, district planning and decentralization were important items on the agenda, which contributed to a greater appreciation of the need for any HIS to have district-level analytic capacities. As decentralization lost priority and district planning was trivialized, a parallel development was that facilities could now report directly into the national web portal. The loss in political priority of decentralization as an objective, along with other social and political factors, contributed to this increased central focus.

Universal health coverage promises to bring in many new institutions, including those related to HIS. One of these would be of output-based resource allocations to facilities, including numbers of cases seen, disease-groups treated, and quality of care rendered. This will be quite different from earlier institutions when budget allocations to facilities were fixed on some normative principle that did not alter with outputs or performance. In such contexts, data collection and measurement of facility performance were given less importance. Higher workloads, reflected through monthly reports, did not bring in more money, and lower workloads did not involve a re-allocation of resources. But in Thailand, where payment for outpatient care is capitation based, each facility— and over 95 per cent of them are public—has to record the number of families registered with it for primary healthcare and report it to get a corresponding allocation. This also means that there exist robust denominators for calculating rates for any subunit. For inpatients, payments in Thailand are made by numbers treated for each disease-related group. South Africa also has a similar system, but going further, since a considerable proportion of resources are allocated based on outputs, there is accountability to the office of the Auditor General. This office, which usually limits itself to auditing finances, now audits the quality of routine health information. The health department, in anticipation of the Auditor General's audit, conducts internal audits of data quality in every district of South Africa, with positive impacts on data quality and use.

Developed nations where IT systems were set up to facilitate claims processing for insurance may not face these problems, thus providing good quality data on outpatient visits, inpatient visits, quality of care, and disease profiles.

In most LMICs, on the other hand, HMIS were established as part of vertical single focus interventions—like malaria control, tuberculosis control, immunization, maternal care—with rigidly defined targets and protocols for use and little space for deviation. The only need for these systems is for monitoring and accountability. This provides an impetus to promote false reporting and to inflate number of cases seen, but not to improve quality of care. In such a context, it becomes natural that data is perceived as something to be passed up passively with least intervention and thought— as is necessary for being held accountable.

The current trends of integration in HMIS influence the volume of information collected and the diversity of sources. This challenges the previously existing sole authority of the programme officer who was responsible for his/her vertical programme—including data collection from subordinate officers in the chain of command, its aggregation, and its truthful reporting. In the earlier vertical design, there was only one version of the truth as far as the programme went—and that was pronounced by the programme officer. In parallel, the statistical officer would have additional command over the population-based survey, and provided an alternative version of the truth versus that of the programme officer—but once in about five years. The problem was that these two versions could be widely different; for example, the programme officer reported a 100 per cent immunization rate, while the external survey put it at 50 per cent, with limited possibilities to understand the source of divergence. It was expected that once HMIS was in place, it could locate the source of such errors in the programme officers' reports and fix it—and this would lead to constructing only one version of the truth. And yes, and that was the aspiration, henceforth it would be the statistician, thanks to the credibility of his office, who would pronounce it.

As web-based online systems multiply, more information becomes visible with the promise of increased transparency. Simultaneously, as the number of surveys increase, the 'single version of the truth' becomes even more difficult to obtain. One solution to this is to design one system onto which everyone reports and to shut down all other systems. The corollary of this demand is to declare one person or office as the final authority with powers to pronounce the truth, and discourage other sources of pronouncements.

The "single window of truth" has proven difficult to achieve as existing systems fight hard to retain their existence. The single window seeks to establish a single authority with a sense of power and control over others with respect to what is the official vesion of the truth, and undermines the power that multiple programmes had hitherto. To subvert this imposition, vertical programmes could create feeder systems and put a version of their data in them. Further, this 'single version' requires protocols for data comparison and error management, and audit trails for tracking what changes are made to the data, where, and by whom. However, these protocols, which represent institutional rules, are never made, and the 'final' version of the truth is subject to continued changes even a few years after closure. Many other sources not under the control of the single authority speak up, and sometimes they become the scoop for journalists and researchers to highlight these issues.

The proof of the pudding is in the eating. Today in a few nations like South Africa and Thailand, information from HMIS has become the main source of actionable information at different administrative levels. Surveys exist to complement the HMIS and to validate it, rather than replace it. In other nations, HMIS exists, but policy and decision-making rests almost exclusively on population-based surveys.

6.3.5 The logic of donor institutions

Donor institutions are important actors in the organizational field that shape influences on HIS reforms in many LMICs. In these countries, the establishment of HMIS, including technical assistance, infrastructure, software, and expertise, is financed by external aid, and is significantly shaped by the perceptions and priorities of donor agencies. Donor agencies are firstly agents for their respective governments and parliaments, which represent the principal and which lay down the policies and procedures to be implemented in countries. At another level, these donor agencies in particular countries serve as principals by virtue of the financial assistance they provide to the countries that may be viewed as agents. The nature of this principal–agent relation and the underlying power relationships are a function of various factors, such as the percentage of donor contribution to a country's national health budget, the respective government's political priorities, and what particular diseases it seeks to support.

There are many reasons for this principal role of the donor agencies in the countries they support. One important reason is that in the theory of health sector reforms that informs most donor agencies, enhanced monitoring is one of the most important routes to ensuring accountability of the LMICs against the financial assistance that they receive. And accountability is usually one of the cardinal objectives of reform with respect to public sector functioning. In institutional analysis, exit, voice, and hierarchy are the three pathways to ensuring accountability. Exit means that consumers have an option to exit public services, given that there are affordable private alternatives possible. But in practice, the latter is difficult to ensure. Voice refers to the ability of communities and individuals to protest—or at least register a grievance and have it redressed immediately. With so many gaps in policy and so many failures in implementation at higher levels, and in a context of under-investment, few governments would encourage protest against themselves. The third, hierarchy, refers to supervision down a chain of command, the strengthening of which, using ICTs, is possible and desirable to both funding agencies and governments. For these reasons, funding the HMIS is a feature of almost every single reform.

Since donor agencies are also answerable to their constituencies back home, they need to be able to assure themselves that there are no leakages of the aid funds they are providing. HMIS is perceived as helping in this process of blocking leakage. The logic of result-based financing, a current priority of donor institutions, is a key reform measure to strengthen HMIS, and requires a strengthened support for its effective implementation. In many nations, external aid is becoming a small, almost insignificant part of all public health expenditure, and positioning this aid in technical assistance for monitoring provides such funding a better 'value for money' proposition than many other alternatives. Given the considerable constraints that governments have in procuring IT services for sustained long-term support with treasury funds, if this process is taken over by donor agencies, it makes things easier for the government to deal with procurement.

Such donor- and external aid-financed HMIS initiatives create, at the highest level, another layer of decision makers that act from a different vantage point than the government given their different principals, and this brings in another diverse set of considerations. For example, the multiple parallel HMIS linked to each vertical programme (e.g. HIV, TB, immunization, etc.) arises from the fact that different donors support each of these verticals through the provision of funds, software, technical assistance, capacity building, and advice. Problems arise when a work has to be certified as completed and the user-client is different from the payer-client. The systems vendor has only to establish to the payer-client that he has done his job, and any lack of performance of the system is because of unrelated institutional problems that the user-client is facing. This is not very difficult to establish. Procurement policies are also not tailored to sustaining, much less continually evolving the system after the project period is over. Hence as projects end, the systems-support donors offer also comes to an end, with no local institutional capacity in place for sustaining and building upon existing systems.

Historically, there are fears in LMICs that donors will give them systems based on theories, standards, and design blueprints derived in Western contexts—which may or may not be appropriate to their needs. However this is not the way donor agencies perceive it. As international experience accumulates, some donor agencies and some nations have come to recognize these problems of procurement, and they see their role to include convincing the aid recipients of the need for institutional changes for procuring, supporting, and deploying IT systems.

If we take DHIS 2 as an example of these changing trends, one interesting development worth noting is in the emerging model of donor support to DHIS 2, which over time has gained acceptance as a solution that is better placed to address many of these issues. Firstly, a multiparty support has emerged with various large bilateral and multilateral donors such as NORAD, Global Fund, WHO, PEPFAR, UNICEF, and others coming together to support University of Oslo to develop and evolve the DHIS 2 core to support priority activities across variety of organizations and countries. This has helped to develop economies of scale, optimize use of resources in its development, and keep it agile and evolving. Secondly the DHIS 2 is now recommended by various global agencies as the platform of choice for HMIS strengthening activities, where technical support and capacity building is easier to organize. DHIS 2 is also projected as a national data warehouse that can accommodate several health programmes, rather than a single one, which allows for integrated thinking and action. A corollary of such decisions regarding DHIS 2 and other open source systems like Open MRS requires acknowledgement of the role of system evolution, capacity building, open source and open standards, and cooperative models of collaboration with a broad base of a number of universities and NGOs in the north and the south—and making institutional changes that can allow these processes to happen.

These institutional changes around DHIS 2 are constantly evolving, developing freely at multiple sites by multiple developers working collaboratively instead of competitively. Though they represent only a small fraction of global HMIS strengthening efforts, they are significant as the supporting concepts are spreading fast. This potentially provides an alternative model to proprietary vendor-based systems' development efforts, which have plagued HMIS strengthening efforts globally for more than three decades.

6.4 **Design Principles for Building Institutions to Support Expanded PHI**

The impact of ICTs is greatly influenced by the institutional context of their introduction and use. Where there are deep flaws in the health sector architecture and programme design, these undermine the effectiveness of the HIS deployed and these design flaws tend to be amplified when they are automated. However if one is conscious of these flaws, and ICTs are designed to address these, ICTs can be a game changer in correcting the structural flaws of health systems and programmes. Some design principles to enable this are elaborated upon next.

6.4.1 Treat information and communications technologies' introduction and use as a process of negotiation

No institutional entity should be powerful enough to impose a solution all on their own, and expect all others to drop their systems and accept their single window of truth. There will never be any single version of the truth and such a quest may not even be desirable. What is needed is a consensus for action, guided by an increasing appreciation of all the evidence and information available. Understanding the terms under which information is produced, disseminated, and used helps to build a better appreciation of the information itself, and make more informed choices of what sources to rely on and for what purposes. Institutional leaderships should shape the change in a more productive direction, and create the environment in which negotiations can take place and consensus decisions can be made.

6.4.2 Enable incentives from the system for all

All stakeholders down the value chain have to be taken on board and should benefit directly from the system. Given the importance of primary data collection, additional importance needs to be given to how the system would benefit the service providers, facility managers, and mid-level managers in terms of new functionalities for use and reduced burden of work related to data collection.

6.4.3 Redefine rules of procurement

The rules of contracting and procurement in Ministries of Health represent deep-rooted institutions which are difficult to change, and adversely impact the nature of new systems that can be introduced. These institutions need to be modified to provide space for open source solutions and standards, encourage small and niche players which may provide better products for lower costs, bring in stronger domain knowledge of public health and systems development, and enable effective support and investment in long-term capacity building initiatives.

6.4.4 Decentralized systems are more effective than centralized ones

Health systems that are decentralized adaptive learning systems are more successful than centralized rigid hierarchical systems. The more decentralized and adaptive a system is, the greater is its potential for learning, and the more likely it is to make use of information.

The reverse may turn out to be true as well—that centralized health systems that make better use of information and have information systems better designed to support use of information will, over time, become more decentralized, adaptive, and learning—and therefore achieve better performance.

6.5 **References**

Braa, J. and Sahay, S. (2012). Health information systems programme—participatory design within the HISP network. In: Simonsen, J. and Robertson, T. (eds.). *Routledge International Handbook of Participatory Design*. Routledge, Abingdon, UK.

Fogel, R.W. and North, D.C (1993). *Economic Performance Through Time, The Sveriges Riksbank Prize in Economic Sciences in Memory of Alfred Nobel 1993, Prize Lecture.* Available at: http://www.nobelprize.org/nobel_prizes/economic-sciences/laureates/1993/ north-lecture.html

North, D.C. (1990). *Institutions, Institutional Change and Economic Performance.* Cambridge University Press, Cambridge, UK.

Ostrom, E. (2011). Background on the institutional analysis and development framework. *Policy Studies Journal*, **39**(1), 7–27.

Piotti, B., Chilundo, B., and Sahay, S. (2006). An institutional perspective on health sector reforms and the process of reframing health information systems case study from Mozambique. *The Journal of Applied Behavioral Science*, **42**(1), 91–109.

Sahay, S., Sæbø, J.I., Mekonnen, S.M., and Gizaw, A.A. (2010). Interplay of institutional logics and implications for deinstitutionalization: case study of HMIS implementation in Tajikistan. *Information Technologies & International Development*, **6**(3), 19.

Weber, M. (1946). Bureaucracy. *From Max Weber: essays in sociology*, 196–244.

Chapter 7

Complexity and Public Health Informatics in Low and Middle-Income Countries

7.1 **Defining Complexity**

Information and communications technologies (ICT) solutions in healthcare are becoming increasingly complex, interdependent, and large scale. Rapid changes in both the landscape of healthcare, with its increasing sophistication and number of services, and in the supporting ICTs, which are becoming internet, devices and cloud-based, are driving this development towards higher levels of complexity. The rapid scale-up of the internet and the mobile networks in low and middle-income countries (LMICs), and their combination—internet over the mobile network—have given health workers and communities access to the internet, even in the remote rural settings of LMICs. This vast and far-reaching new internet and cloud-based infrastructure is providing an electronic platform for the rapid scaling of ICTs in reach, as well as in scope and size. Health workers even in remote communities are becoming connected to the internet, using and getting familiarized with Google and social media platforms such as Facebook and WhatsApp. Given the enabling cloud-based infrastructure, the number and types of ICT solutions are rapidly growing and systems and data are increasingly being moved to the cloud, and 'big' data, as discussed in Chapter 5, is becoming the new paradigm. The increasing number of systems is followed by an increasing need for their integration, as the services they are reflecting have high levels of interdependencies. While the cloud and the internet provide a better platform for networking and interoperability between systems than did the 'old' stand-alone systems, the process of moving data and systems to the cloud as such is not leading to integration and it is, in most cases, only replicating the previous fragmentation with more data and technical sophistication.

Fragmentation and complexity of systems are two terms that are sometimes used interchangeably, but here we will emphasize an important difference. While fragmentation may be understood as a bit destructive in the context of health information systems (HIS), with systems being broken into small or separate and uncoordinated parts, complexity is a term used to denote that systems consist of many different parts that interact in multiple ways, such that the whole system seems to be evolving on its own. While the term *fragmentation* is referring to a lack of interaction and coordination, complexity may be seen as having a focus on the potential and actual interaction, both intended and unintended, between the different parts of an overall system. Complexity is therefore useful as a perspective to understand HIS and ICTs in the age of the internet, where systems have inherently increased interdependencies. In this chapter, we discuss different aspects of complexity and provide a model which helps provide a perspective to understand Expanded PHIs. The model conceptualizes complexity along the two dimensions of systems: being more or less networked, and, being more or less characterized by uncertainty as to the context of use.

Furthermore, we discuss strategies to manage complexity using the concept of 'attractor for change' (Plsek and Wilson 2001) from the field of complex adaptive systems (CAS). We conceptualize HIS as socio-technical systems where cultivation is suggested as a strategy for creating attractors for change and complex HIS.

7.1.1 Understanding complexity in low and middle-income countries

One key objective in this chapter is the development of a model for understanding and analysing complexity in public health informatics in LMICs, and the various arguments leading up to this model. The level of formalization of business processes is an example of an important dimension to apply when analysing complexity. In LMICs, the informal sector of the economy will typically be bigger than the formal sector. This informal-formal dichotomy is replicated in many aspects of society and develops as part of the general process of modernization, as the organization of work gets more formalized and rule-based. Computers are 'dumb' and only the absolute formalized and structured aspects of work and business processes can be successfully computerized. Limited formalization and standardization means that interaction between the various components of the complex system, that is between business processes and organizational structures in health, will be more informal, less standardized and rule-based, and consequently more 'complex' to computerize. The meaning and handling of complexity in LMICs may therefore be different than in more thoroughly modernized countries. We illustrate this aspect of complexity in LMICs with an example from an Asian country, where the computerization of the licensing of health workers faced the problem of a mismatch between regulation (formal and detailed requirements) and how the regulation was practised (the required categories of courses, for example, did not exist)—which was much more informal than the prescribed procedures.

Hans Rosling raised a similar point at the Global Health summit in Washington DC (June 2015) that the World Health Organization (WHO) strategy of establishing birth and death registration in all countries was doomed to failure in a number of LMICs. This process had taken more than 200 years in Sweden, and many countries would not be ready for implementing this programme due to the state of the processes of modernization and formalization for the various institutions involved. Uncertainty regarding the quality of health data—and more generally of population-based data, such as the lack of reliable census data, is linked to similar aspects of poorly developed institutions, and the heightened complexity in getting reliable estimates.

We first discuss fragmentation of HIS and present a theoretical framework using complexity to understand it, drawing upon concepts of attractors for change drawn from CAS. In discussing strategies for addressing complexity, we take the notion of cultivation from information systems research and illustrate this analysis approach by drawing upon the case of the dashboard in Indonesia. Furthermore, we present a different integration approach based on a data warehouse in Ghana. Both of these cases illustrate aspects of complexity arising from the mismatch between regulation and practice in a LMIC. These different examples help to develop a model for analysing complexity. Finally, we conclude with strategies for developing systems and handling complexity in LMICs.

7.2 Complexity and Fragmentation in Health Information Systems

Looking at the history of HIS in LMICs, increasing fragmentation, lack of shared standards, and poor coordination have been seen as the major challenges. In particular, since the advent of the large HIV/AIDS programmes around 2000, the tendency has been that more and more NGOs, donors, and projects have established their own parallel reporting structures greatly magnifying fragmentation. A focus on HIV/AIDS patients and expensive antiretroviral drugs made the ability to track patients and manage clinical pathways increasingly important, which again led to a proliferation of patient record systems alongside an increasing number of typically overlapping aggregate data reporting systems at the facility level. To be able to manage these big programmes' effective integration with the general health services will require quality data, both from population and clinical care contexts.

A key challenge in this landscape of fragmented systems is the quest for integration, not only of the health service and population-based 'HMIS' and 'M&E'-like systems, but also of patient-based and population-based health data and systems. Population and patient-based systems have historically evolved independently of each other, are based on different logics, and are being developed and promoted by different communities with different cultures of action. In order to be able to provide integrated information support to health systems across multiple levels of management and governance, these systems and communities need to interoperate within themselves, as also with other systems and communities, such as those for human resources, drugs and logistics, transport, insurance, finance, and many others.

Integration of HIS has been on the global agenda for a long time, but during the last few years, the situation has started to change. Led by WHO, big donor organizations are now increasingly demanding the integration of data and systems. These changes in attitudes are welcome and are being expressed at a time when the rapid spread of the internet has in fact made it easier than before. We can say we are moving from the challenge of handling fragmentation to that of handling the complexity of systems.

7.2.1 Analytical concepts

Complexity refers to a situation, or an overall system, where many different parts are interacting in multiple ways, so that the whole system appears to be evolving on its own. It can be a big city, a beehive, or the internet. CAS is a field within complexity science which studies the adaptation dynamics of complex systems: how different parts of the system and their interaction adapt and evolve to changing conditions. CAS pays particular attention to the study of how order emerges, rather than being created through design. Central to the emergence of orders is the notion of attractors. A typical example of an attractor is a shared standard that is followed by many. For example, MS Windows, for good or for bad, created order in the personal computing area. The creation of 'attractors for change' (Plsek and Wilson 2001) may be used as a strategy to bring about changes in areas with limited agreement, standards, and stability, such as fragmented HIS. Scaling is another central concept in complexity science, which is a useful lens to understand how this emerging order can expand.

> 'Complex, adaptive systems exhibit coherence through scaling and self-similarity. Scaling is the property of complex systems in which one part of the system reproduces the same structure and patterns that appear in other parts of the system'
>
> (Eoyang 1996, p. 36).

The example of broccoli is a metaphor to understand scaling in a natural system, where branches and sub-branches replicate the structure of the whole plant. However, information systems are inherently social systems, and cannot be represented through the broccoli metaphor, as people and organizations are always context specific (Braa *et al.* 2007). In their web models, Kling and Scacchi (1982), give a theoretical framework to understand why and how large information systems tend to be tied to the social context through a complex web of associations, as contrasted with the discrete-entity model view of information systems being socially neutral technical systems.

> 'When an analyst uses a discrete-entity model to understand the computing capabilities of an organisation he usually begins by asking, "What kind of equipment and facility do they have?" In contrast, analysts using a web model begin by asking: "What kinds of things do people do here?"'

(Kling and Scacchi 1982, p. 9).

The web model emphasizes historical legacy and context in system development:

> 'Since information systems are bound up with the infrastructures available, and since these evolve over time, computing developments are shaped by a set of historical commitments. In short, web models view computing developments as complex social objects constrained by their context, infrastructure and history'

(Kling and Scacchi 1982, p. 69).

The other relevant concept for understanding HIS is of cultivation, which denotes a way of shaping technology based on resources and potential already present, which is fundamentally different from construction as an engineering method based on structured planning which assumes a clean slate (Dahlbom and Janlert 1996). As the metaphor indicates, cultivation is about interfering with, supporting, and controlling natural processes that are already there, as in nurturing and watering a plant to nurture an 'organism' with a life of their own (Ciborra 1997). As a strategy in systems development and design, cultivation is thus seen as in opposition to structured methods and consisting of incremental and evolutionary approaches, and 'piecemeal engineering' (Popper 1986). While cultivation represents an approach within the social system model, structured engineering methods are linked to the discrete-entity model.

We illustrate this approach where attractors cultivate change as a way of addressing complexity with an example from Indonesia, as featured in Case Study 7.1.

(continued on page 161)

Case Study 7.1 Indonesia: DHIS 2 Dashboard as an 'Attractor for Change'

Indonesia is a large country with the fourth largest population in the world, with a well- developed infrastructure showing some regional variations. In terms of HIS, the country is fairly typical; while a number of vertical health programme-specific systems have moved to the cloud and the amount of data have increased, the systems remain as separate silos with little to no sharing of data. In this case, we describe a newly initiated process under the leadership of the MoH to develop an integrated dashboard for the sharing of data across health programmes and systems, starting from a point where no shared standards existed. All systems are, for example, using different codes for health facilities, making it impossible to share or compare data at that level. This agreement to work together on the process of integrating their systems is, on the one hand, based on a genuine need for shared information and a shared 'trust' in the dashboard concept. The dashboard is understood as an achievable approach for integration without disturbing the underlying systems too much, or without too high a cost. We'll use the dashboard as an 'attractor for change' concept to analyse the case.

Indonesia has a strong federal structure where provinces and districts manage their own health services and budgets relatively independent from the national MoH. There are stark contrasts between the developed western part of the country (Java, Bali, Sumatra) and the much less developed eastern parts (Papua). In Java island, all health centres (called 'Puskesmas') have electronic patient record systems, very often locally developed, and often of different types even within the same district. At the national level, health programmes have their own systems, many of them web-based (e.g. TB, HIV/AIDS), but also Excel-based (e.g. malaria). Data from the health centres are reported to the districts, where it is then compiled and captured in national systems. The HIV/AIDS system for example, runs patient-based systems at the health centre level and reports aggregate data to the district where it is captured in the national system. All programmes have their officers at the district level who process data for sending onto the province and national levels. However, despite all data passing through the districts, there is no shared data repository.

The national level is running a system called KOMDAT, which collects data for about 130 national health indicators, based on data aggregated by district. In addition, the recently established universal health insurance agency (BPJS) has established a patient-based insurance system in all hospitals and gradually all health centres. A key problem identified is that at no level is any systematic overview provided of the integrated data across health programmes, administrative levels, and health services. For example, when visiting Malang district, we saw the only way to get an overview of data was to meet the officer in charge of each programme; a situation repeated at the province and national levels. The one system trying to address this need is the KOMDAT, but since it is based on data aggregated by district, there is no way to check data quality at the facility level, and the system is therefore not trusted by the administrators.

We provide below our conceptualization of the HIS and its underlying complexity in Figure 7.1.

The situation differs between districts. For example, in Surabaya City they have developed a comprehensive patient-based system covering all programmes and health facilities. In all districts in Yogyakarta province, every health centre has its own electronic patient record system to report patient data to the district, where aggregated district reports are generated. In contrast, in Malang district, there is a plethora of systems in use at the facility level and limited integration at the district level. Data are, however, reported from facilities on paper and in some cases MS Excel (e.g. for immunization), and compiled as district Excel sheets with data

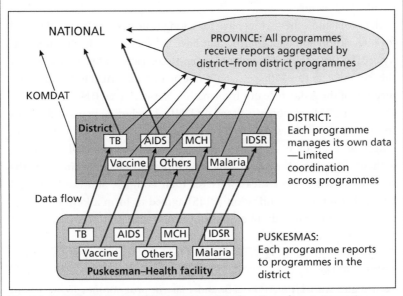

Fig. 7.1 Complexity as seen in Indonesia's HIS before the reform intervention.

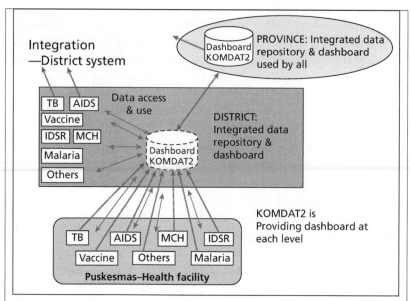

Fig. 7.2 Proposed integration model using DHIS 2.

by facility. When reporting to province, however, data are aggregated by districts. The district is the only place where data by facility may be found, while the province only has data by districts, available in Excel sheets in email attachments.

The MoH and other actors have for a long time acknowledged the need for integration and data sharing, but have believed—due to the complexity arising from the independence given to districts and provinces under the federal structure—that it would not be possible. At the third general meeting of the Asian eHealth Information Network (AeHIN) in Manila in December 2014, dashboards based on DHIS 2 including maps and graphs from several countries such as Bangladesh and Laos were demonstrated, reflecting a proof of concept of what could be realistically achieved without disturbing the underlying structures too much. Seeing this, the Indonesian team saw its feasibility for their country, and the MoH and national insurance organization (BPJS) agreed to form a joint project to develop an integrated dashboard using the DHIS 2 platform (see Fig. 7.2 for the proposed model).

A proposal for funding was submitted to the Global Fund and accepted, and the project started in 2015. During the initial work, agreements have been made with HIV/AIDS, TB, and malaria programmes to start with importing their data into the DHIS 2 data warehouse, to be used for visu-alizations through the dashboard. In parallel, work has started with BPJS, where the data structures are more complex, and cannot be imported directly into the data warehouse. A first step for this integration is to develop a facil-ity register where facility IDs used by the different systems can be mapped to a common reference.

The project seeks to manage complexity by creating integrated dash-boards in Indonesia, but it is still early days to produce tangible results. Some systems have completely moved to the warehouse, others have held out and continue stand-alone, while others are making the change partially and gradually. However, the interesting aspect here is that the 'dashboard' has started to emerge as an 'attractor for change', with the different stake-holders converging around it to discuss, practice, and visualize change.

In the next case study (7.2), we discuss another example of attractors of change and the cultivation of change in another context—the implemen-tation of the District Health Information Management System (DHIMS) in Ghana.

7.3 Informality and Fuzzy Complexity in Public Health Information Systems and Low and Middle-Income Countries

In this section, we discuss how computerization is historically based on long-term structuring of processes of formalization and institutional development. We argue that complexity is linked to levels of formalization, and low levels of formalization, such as in public health in LMICs, are characterized by high levels of complexity and uncertainty.

7.3.1 Formalization and general development

Computerization typically takes place within formalized and closed domains, where the programmer selects which objects and their properties are needed in order to perform a particular task. ICT development builds on historical pro-cesses of formalization in society (Jervell 1991; Greenbaum 1998; Berg 1997), resulting from a dynamic interplay between the use of formalized and closed descriptions, which contributes to the building of artificial environments, which again make it possible to further formalize and close. Formalization tends to create artificial environments in an otherwise untamed world. In the

(continued on page 164)

Case Study 7.2 Central Server and Scaling in Ghana: Managing Complexity and Creating an 'Attractor in the Cloud'

Ghana implemented a web and central server based data warehouse in 2012 called DHIMS, based on the DHIS 2 platform (Poppe *et al.* 2013). This replaced an earlier MS Office-based proprietary system called DHIMS, implemented in 2008 in all districts and hospitals in the country. Data was submitted on paper forms to the districts where data were captured, checked for quality, and sent to the province as email attachments, and from there to the national level. The decision to go for DHIS 2 on a central server solution was taken, first of all, because internet had reached all districts and the MoH wanted to go 'online', and wanted to adopt an open source approach.

From a Stand-Alone System to Central Server and the Cloud

During the DHIMS pilot phase (2004–2007), health programmes and other actors were mobilized to agree on a shared set of data sets and reporting formats. This process was successful, and by 2008 all reporting forms from most health programmes were unified in one compilation of forms included in the DHIMS software. Despite this initial success, however, what happened after is quite typical. The software used to capture and manage these integrated data forms was developed by a private company and the source code was retained by them. The software was never fully finished, and as funds ran out the company did not continue without payment. With changes in requirements, and a stagnant software, health programmes started to develop their own reporting mechanisms, mostly low-scale systems in Excel. The Reproductive and Child Health (RCH) unit received big funding from the Global Fund and used it to develop their own application, creating a conflict in the previously unified process. This process was subsequently abandoned. Seeing this situation, the Ghana Health Service contracted another company to fix the existing software bugs, and the discrepancy between the programmes' requirements and the DHIMS increased. Without the source code and adequate documentation about the different tables and their relations, the bugs could not be fixed, and the existing data was lost.

This overall deterioration of the situation spurred the Ghana Health Service and all health programmes to collaborate on a new initiative to unify all reporting formats based on the DHIS 2, but the system was called DHIMS 2 to show continuity with the past. System customization, supported by the University of Oslo team, started in 2011, followed by training in the facilities and a roll-out based on a relative low-key budget and without prior piloting. The system and the internet were tested and they worked, and in April 2012, the old system was abandoned and the new system was implemented. The changeover went smoothly using the existing infrastructure. With an internet web-based system, rollout at a national scale was primarily about investing in training and human capacity development, rather than in machines. The rapid rollout and the immediate availability of data impressed all stakeholders, and arguably an 'attractor in the cloud was created', which gradually mobilized more health programmes to give up their vertical reporting and join the DHIMS 2 process. The cloud could serve as an attractor, as one only one instance of the DHIMS 2 could be accessed by all the users, and all updates, and bug fixing could be carried out at one place which was instantly reflected to all users. This is in contrast to the earlier rather stagnant system, when bug fixes and system updates were carried out in each site of use. This is also in contrast to earlier changes, when all existing systems have to be dropped when a new one arrives. In this approach, existing systems could align and gradually evolve, and then link up with increasing effectiveness over time.

Data Quality and Data Access in the New System

A study carried out in 2014 demonstrated a significant improvement of data quality (Adaletey *et al.* 2014), with 88 per cent reporting completeness. Contributing to this improvement was the new practice of peer review of data by districts at regional meetings, which again was made possible by the fact that all data was real time and accessible over the web. The increased and immediate visibility of all data spurred on data quality improvements.

All health facilities and budget management centres are expected to account for their stewardship at biannual and annual reviews, where performance is seen in relation to annual plans and targets achieved over the period. This is done at various levels through a series of regional and divisional presentations. From 2013, it has been instructed that data from the DHIS 2 should be used for peer-performance review, which has created a significant focus on data and data quality throughout the entire organization. Regional directors are expected by their superiors to show 100 per cent reporting rates from their districts. Maybe the biggest change with the new system is that now everybody can access their data online, whereas before, data was in the custody of the health information system officers who served as the gatekeepers and could no longer argue that 'data was not yet ready for distribution'. In contrast, now data could be accessed 'as is', even prior to its cleaning. This easy access to data at local levels is an interesting development in relation to our discussion on the hypothesis of losing local control in the cloud-based infrastructure. In Ghana, more people at the local level have access to the data online than before in the local systems.

DHIMS 2 as Attractor for Change

As the DHIMS 2 scaled, it emerged as a central attractor for change, and gradually most other health programmes joined the process: clinical services, case-based mortality reporting, laboratories, stock control, disease control, TB, EPI, and malaria. The HIV/AIDS programme is currently working to become part of the overall DHIMS 2 framework. We may summarize that the cloud-based DHIMS 2 implementation created an attractor that convinced the various actors, from the general director to all health programmes, to align, evolve, and over time link up, which over a few years contributed to the materialization of an integrated reporting framework. This deployment of the cloud infrastructure offered through the 'Platform as a Service' model helped the move from multiple MS Office Access-based installations in all districts to one central server, also leading to strengthened support mechanisms and improved use. But typical of complex adaptive systems, as one problem gets solved, others emerge. One emerging challenge is the need for a new kind of 'higher' level technical expertise of server and system administration required than what was needed by MS Office systems, which was also more readily available in Ghana. To fill this capacity gap, the Ghana Health Service is currently depending on external support from the University of Oslo, but this tends to shift control back to the central level—representing a change in the opposite direction from local control, which was the desired end. There is thus an inherent dialectic in complex systems—some changes are predictable and some are not, some are desirable, and some are not—but advance only takes place on such terms.

developed systems which have a higher level of formalization inherent, the degree of artificiality will be lower as compared to LMICs.

> 'Without this formalization there would have been practically no arithmetical calculations, text processing and book keeping to be done on the computers'

(Jervell 1991, p. 176).

An example: In an Asian country, the Ministry of Health (MoH) is developing a system consisting of multiple parts for the licensing of health workers and health facilities, lodging of complaints over treatment from the public, and other aspects of patient security. This requires various standards which are yet to be developed. For example, licensed health workers are required to take an accredited 48-hour course at an approved institution, and without it, their licence will be revoked. The problem is that there are too few approved institutions and courses, limiting the ability to grant and revoke licences. The development of a computer-based system to support the continuous education part of the licensing system encountered a general problem when trying to computerize existing informal processes and its attendant lack of standards and regulation. This makes it difficult to develop the system. Of course, the system can be designed to accept any course, as is the practice today, but that in reality will mean that it is accepted that the law is not followed. The important point made is that the introduction of a computer system into an informal process, which in fact was breaking the law, represents a breakdown of the current practice because the shortcoming and lack of the law—in this case standardized courses—becomes evident for everybody to see. Formalization and standardization, which are part of historical processes, have been going on longer and wider in industrialized countries than in LMICs. The development of ICTs in LMICs is therefore characterized with a higher level of uncertainty than experienced in industrialized countries.

In section 7.3.2 we see similar differences between hospital and clinical HISs and population-based HISs, making their integration a challenging task.

7.3.2 **Formalization in medicine and public health**

Foucault (1975) shows in *The Birth of the Clinic* that the arrival of hospitals in the period 1780–1840 affected the way diseases were understood, and a precise language for describing and handling diseases was then developed. Industrialization—with its demand for labour and a healthy population—led to the reorganization of the hospitals, from places to hide away the sick, to curing-machines for industrial work. This led to a redefinition of medical practice:

> ' ... the space of the hospital must be organised according to a concrete therapeutic strategy, through the uninterrupted presence of hierarchical prerogatives of doctors, through systems of observations, notation and record-taking, which make it possible to fix a knowledge of different cases, to follow their particular evolution, and also to globalise the data which bear on the long-term life as a whole population ... '
>
> (Foucault 1975).

The arrival of the hospital led to a spiral of developments and institutionalization within the health profession, along with the standardization of medical education, knowledge and practice (Kirkebøen 1993). The formalization, standardization, and closed descriptions enabled computerization of patient records, forms, registers, and the various events associated with them like procedures, laboratory tests, and surgeries. The ICD (International Classification of Diseases) administered by the WHO is both a result and a cause of healthcare formalization and standardization. ICD is more than a hundred years old and has been revised about every 10 years since the end of the nineteenth century. While historically HIS have focused on hospitals and formalized procedures (Rodrigues and Israel 1995), the public health approach focuses on what is going on in the community, which is less formalized and plays out in a more open setting.

An example of a typically formalized and closed problem area is a patient database covering those who have been served by a facility. A less formalized area is a similar register of children who have not completed their immunization scheme in a community, or a register of pregnant women due for their first antenatal care (ANC) visit. While the hospital HIS focuses on what is going on within their walls and is registering those who are passing through the doors, the public health HIS, in principle, focuses on what is going on in the community and in the population at large, which by definition is an 'open' area. It is difficult to establish good public health and population-based HISs that produce quality data. However, despite good intentions and advanced technologies, there will always be a certain level of uncertainty linked to population-based data. To link back to our topic of complexity, we could say that public health and population-based HISs are more complex than clinically-based HIS, because their linkages to the real world (population) are characterized with more uncertainty and fuzziness. However, HIS in hospitals are also regarded as being complex because of their numerous 'moving' parts that need to interact with other hospital systems; for example, drugs, insurance, and diets. It is not fruitful, then, to say that population-based systems are more, or less, complex than clinical systems, but to recognize the differences in complexity. The intersection between clinical systems and public health systems itself represents an interesting area of complexity.

Systems based on computerized medical records are often claimed to be more accurate than traditional paper-based data collection. Anecdotal evidence tells us that this is not necessarily the case. During a study in 2003 of HIS in the South African Limpopo province, one of the authors met with the health information officer involved in a medical record hospital project covering all hospitals in the province. He was told that the data on outpatient cases were so poor that they could not be used and they relied on the traditional paper-based health management information systems (HMIS) instead. The indicated reason for this was that in a lot of the cases, that is, the paper patient folders due for data capturing, were 'piling up and not captured' due to a lack of manpower, as well as the poor trust of the medical personnel in the system. A medical record project conducted more recently in Rwanda from 2008 reports a similar outcome. When data from the medical record pilot were compared with the national HMIS system, the ANC numbers differed. Also, not all cases in this instance were captured in the medical record system and the paper-based HMIS data was more complete. In both cases of South Africa and Rwanda, the medical record systems were not well-tuned with the social system including the work practices and behaviour of the health workers and patients, and this alignment was better with the routine HMIS. It is not evident that by extending the medical records system to the area of public health that data quality will automatically improve; indeed, it is possible that new complexities will be encountered. In most LMICs, recording continues on paper and this is the basis of use by the data collector who is also a provider, while reporting happens onto a digital system and the data thus reported is lost to local use. But where recording is brought onto digital platforms, the complexities do not diminish—but they are significantly redefined.

7.3.3 Data quality and population-based systems

In 2008, there was a big dispute about the quality of immunization data reported from LMICs and used by GAVI (The Vaccine Alliance) for remuneration of performance. A study comparing data from household surveys and official MoH statistics from 1986 to 2006 in 193 countries, showed that data from most of the 51 countries eligible for GAVI support were inflated and that the immunization coverages were significantly less than reported (Stephen *et al.* 2008). Since immunization data reported from countries were collected through their HMIS, the study thus provided a general critique of the data quality in these systems. Furthermore, it is argued that the inflated reporting is, to a large extent, due to the incentives provided by GAVI for each additional child fully immunized (USD 20). While there are indeed exceptions, most countries are struggling with data quality from their HMIS. Following the argument made earlier about the relation between complexity and formalization, we argue that this holds for immunization data and GAVI as well. Household surveys were used to establish 'true' numbers of immunized children, which were then compared with official figures found to be 'false'. Without going into the details of the methodology, an important point to note is that household surveys use population censuses in order to estimate country figures. And population census data in LMICs (Africa, in particular) is a much more questionable data source than the routine HMIS data. For example, population censuses in

Nigeria have always been highly disputed and politicized—the current population estimate ranges from 120 to 200 million, with 170 being the consensus. Population in states and local government are translated into budgets and the proportion between the Muslim north and the Christian south translates into politics. The 2006 census 'gave' the north 75 million and the south 65 million. Consequently, the south rejected the numbers and the north endorsed them. The point here is that population-based data need to be understood as also contributing to the fuzziness.

The WHO and other actors acknowledge the problem of population data and have launched a global initiative to strengthen civil registration and vital statistics (CRVS) systems for birth and death registration. As mentioned earlier, Hans Rosling warned against this general strategy and argued that it had taken more than 200 years to achieve universal birth registration in Sweden and that many of the less developed countries in the world were not ready for such systems. Vital registration of births and baptisms, marriages, deaths, and burials became regulated as a church law in Sweden in 1686. From the early 1700s, vital events from the entire country were registered in the church books. Relatively early it was raised as a concern that there was no centralized instruction as to how the books were to be kept, and it was done through many different practices, making it difficult, for example, to keep records of movements across church parishes. From 1860, efforts to standardize record-keeping began, and in 1894 standard forms for church records began to be used countrywide (https://familysearch.org/learn/wiki/en/Sweden_Church_Records) that eventually led to the founding of the modern day Swedish Medical Birth Register in 1973, which includes data on practically all deliveries in Sweden. Interestingly enough, even in Sweden, perceived as one of the most regulated countries in the world, 0.5 to 3 per cent of infants' records are missing completely, and a certain proportion of the records are incomplete (https://www.socialstyrelsen.se/register/halsodataregister/medicinskafodelseregistret/inenglish).

The points of emphasis are that, first, computerization of vital registration in Sweden, and in many countries in Europe, builds upon centuries of processes of establishing regulations, formalization, and standardization. Second, the computerization of 'business' processes, such as universal birth registration, are fraught with problems when they are not formalized—the point argued by Hans Rosling. Since LMICs in general will have larger parts of society which are less formalized, the complexity and challenges encountered in ICT implementation will be greater. LMICs also face large problems of migration and displacement that make population denominators inherently more difficult to measure. Migration is an increasing problem in many developed nations too, but this is largely across national border areas. LMICs are also faced with large internal migrations. In addition, the scale, seasonality, and unpredictability of large movements of people in LMICs enhances complexities for public health informatics in LMICs that we are yet to begin to understand and address. Nor is it only a problem of denominators. One of the great challenges is to provide for continuity of care, and enable case-based follow-up in diseases such as TB and HIV across these movements of people.

There are areas, such as the cloud, where LMICs may be as 'advanced' as the industrialized world. Development is best understood as a dynamic patchwork of areas in different states of maturity, where there is unevenness between areas, sectors, and communities. In some areas, development occurs incrementally as well as in leaps, and in others, development may be retarded. Development is thus not linear, since latecomers may be the first to be developed, and economically developed areas may become deprived. In Galtung's (1971) 'Structural theory of imperialism', the opposition, or mutual duality, between the core and the periphery, or developed and underdeveloped countries, regions, and areas, is replicated recursively within both the core and the periphery. This dynamic relationship is evident in areas of a third world city, where slums are serving developed industrial areas in a mutual relationship. A similar pattern of dichotomy is seen between hospitals and clinical HIS on the one side, and public health and population-based ICTs and HIS on the other. This book tries to focus on understanding these dichotomies (such as lack of trust in data quality) and how to address them. Handling of the complexity of more or less interacting systems and working towards a higher level of integration and coordination in areas of weak formalization will require the application of strategies to handle uncertainty and fuzziness.

7.4 **Models of Complexity, Big Data, and Service**

The internet and cloud computing have brought us Google, Facebook, instant communication, and limitless access to information, but also the possibility for massive surveillance through analysis of big data, as revealed by computer professional and former Central Intelligence Agency (CIA) employee, Edward Snowden. Complexity and big data are among the important consequences of this new era of moving huge amounts of data and systems to the cloud. The challenge of data quality in population-based systems stems from the problem of weak formalization. Next we discuss the implications of the cloud service models regarding the question of who and how to manage big data—can this be done externally by service providers? We shall also refer back to big data and the service models discussed in Chapter 5.

7.4.1 **Big data and service models**

Big data was first described in 2001 as the challenge of increased Volumes, Velocity, and Variety of data, referred to as the 'Three Vs' of Big Data (Laney 2001). Later IBM came up with a fourth 'V'; *Veracity*, which is of particular relevance to us as it refers to the messiness, doubtful quality, or trustworthiness of the data. The bigger, more varied, and complex the data, the less controllable will be its quality and accuracy. The fuzziness and open-ended aspects of data contribute to making its quality an ever-moving target. The dimension of veracity provides a root cause for complexity, providing a key argument for why health data is not likely to become fully outsourced and black-boxed to cloud big data service providers, and why it should remain in local control.

Big data, as discussed in Chapter 5, is a consequence of cloud computing where large amounts of data can be stored at central servers. Cloud computing refers to software hosted on the internet without the user needing to know where it is hosted or how to closely manage it. 'In the cloud' means that data is stored on remote servers and not on local ones, similar to web-based email accounts such as Gmail, Yahoo, Hotmail, and social media applications like Facebook. They are all in the 'cloud', or in fact 'on the ground', in remote servers, locations of which are not known, or need not be known, to the users.

As also discussed in Chapter 5, the cloud infrastructure is typically made available through a variety of 'service' models. The lowest end of the spectrum of service models (called Infrastructure as a Service, or IaaS) is when the vendor owns and manages the hardware; and the organization owns the application, the data, and the various middlewares needed to run the application. This model is, for example, used by many DHIS 2 implementations taking place on Linode or Amazon. Virtual configuration of the server enables its size to grow with demand in an elastic way. Platform as a Service (PaaS) represents the next level of service model where the vendor in addition to the IaaS services, also provides some of the needed support for the application. In the Software as a Service (SaaS) model, the provider manages the application itself. BAO Systems is an example of an organization (based in the United States) which serves as a SaaS provider for DHIS 2. However, comprehensive data warehouse systems for routine HMIS data in countries, such as in the example from Ghana, are closely linked to the country contexts, and metadata and data sets are difficult to manage externally. Analytics as a Service (AaaS) represents the high end of the service models, where the provider seeks to give an end-to-end service, including managing and analysing the data. Several mobile telephone-based systems and service providers in LMICs are providing AaaS as end-to-end systems, from data collection by mobiles to data management and data processing for customers. We give an example of such a mobile-based project later on in this section.

We illustrated the complexity of health systems through the example of a DHIS 2 cloud-based data warehouse deployment in a big African country, Ghana, which had poor infrastructure. DHIS 2 is a platform for building systems responding to a variety of information requirements from health programmes. For each requirement, the details need to be identified and metadata for data elements and indicators designed and created—all within a coherent framework across modules and requirements. The variety of information needs and conditions makes the mapping of the software to both the reality of the health services and the software itself highly complex. Efforts to manage the development and running of DHIS 2 as a 'service' from the outside was tried, but not with success. In one example, data collection forms for a new health programme on TB in a country, which were relatively complex, were sent to an experienced HISP node for building the metadata. Even such a limited task turned out to be quite complex, because questions to the users had to go through the service provider, which was also based outside the country, who then in turn needed to ask somebody in the country, resulting in a long chain of translations and lost meanings, both ways. It turned out that it was very difficult to develop one part of the system without full access to the overall metadata structure. This strategy of step-wise development of the metadata structure and overall system, by different parties, turned out to be very complicated because of the lack of an overall design strategy guided by local knowledge. Poor metadata design caused the system to perform poorly and even to crash, which led to the task of reconfiguring the whole database and system. The server was hosted abroad by an international hosting company, while the MoH wanted national hosting, adding to the challenges. In another example, a third party company was responsible for setting up the DHIS 2 to include data from the broad range of health services. All communication between the MoH and the actual developers was in writing going through the main contractor, and caused misunderstandings, wrong decisions, and delays.

These two brief examples illustrate the need for close collaboration between the users, business analysts, and developers for the building of any HIS. Higher end service models, such as SaaS and AaaS, are detached from local presence and inherent with greater complexity. By design, they are very difficult to make happen.

7.4.2 **A model for analysing complexity**

As a general rule we say that the higher the complexity, the less possible it is to black-box and outsource the system. In the following model, we analyse complexity along two dimensions: more or less context-sensitive, and more or less networked or interdependent of other systems.

The context-sensitive versus context-free dichotomy

Complexity is a function of the nature of interaction of the system with local business processes, their levels of formalization, and the rate of change of the different components. The stronger the interaction and lower the levels of formalization, the more unique features the system will need to include, making it more context-sensitive. This links with the web model (Kling and Scacchi 1982) presented earlier, where the social systems model represents the context-sensitive end of the continuum, and the discrete-entity model, the context-free end.

The more or less networked and interdependent dichotomy

The more networked a system and the more dependent it is on other systems and organizational structures, the higher is the level of complexity, and the less possible it is to black-box and outsource the system. The traditional fragmentation of HIS, where each disease-specific programme makes its own system, is easier to outsource than an integrated system for TB or HIV/AIDS, including co-infections. In Figure 7.3 we illustrate these two dimensions of complexity. Complexity is low when the systems in question are relatively context-free and have low dependencies with other systems. In contrast, complexity is 'very' high when systems are both context-sensitive and have multiple connections and dependencies, and in-between there is a continuum of more or less complexity. The project to develop integrated dashboards in Indonesia illustrates a system of high complexity, both in terms of the numerous connections and

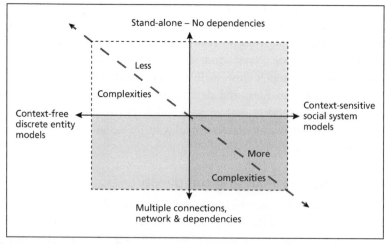

Fig. 7.3 Model of complexity of public health informatics.

interdependencies with specific health programmes' institutional structures, identifiers, and with other context- specific factors.

7.4.3 **Outsourcing of services from the south to the north**

As the cloud-based infrastructure is now global, and also available to the LMICs, one scenario is that service providers in the rich and industrialized countries are taking over the management of systems and data in the least developed countries. The possibility for the remote management of data collection through mobile telephones contributes to the heightened complexity.

The sequence of more and more sophisticated service models, with AaaS as the most advanced, may, by technology optimists (or pessimists), be seen as a transition towards an increasingly 'black-boxed' system of information services. In this scenario, provider companies can potentially take over an ever-increasing part of the HIS, and provide them as services from the rich to the poor countries. This may lead to deskilling and disempowerment in the south. Let's give an example:

Examples from the Gambia and Uganda

Many projects in LMICs are exploring ways of using mobile phones for remote data reporting and communication, and opening up for the new business models of 'software-based services'. What is happening in many countries in Africa now is that international mobile network providers are targeting donor-funded health programmes and projects working in remote areas, and providing end-to-end infrastructure and software solutions for data capture, data management, and analysis at a cost, paid by the rich donor, and typically not integrated within the national HIS framework.

A typical example is a project by Pfizer and Vodafone in the Gambia to monitor stock and distribution of malaria drugs in dispensaries. Vodafone is providing the entire infrastructure—SIM cards if needed (users have their own telephones), mobile network, air time, data management in their 'cloud' and provision of the data to the users. The Vodafone 'cloud' is in London, so everything is located and managed abroad. The web-based national HIS is running on DHIS 2. The national HIS team tried to argue the need for an integrated architecture approach, and suggested to feed the data reported by the Vodafone mobiles into the national HIS, as establishing yet another vertical system would only add to the complexity and wastage of resources. These efforts to integrate the approaches, however, have been in vain. Vodafone argued quite frankly that such integration efforts could only be included 'if there is a place for them in the value chain'.

It is our general view that business models which are locating value chains derived from Africa, outside Africa, are of no use for Africa. But more specifically, outsourcing of what may be labelled the 'ICT learning and innovation chain' from Africa to the West—as illustrated by this case—may be even more harmful. A major problem was that it was not locally run and sustained, but was part of a foreign company's 'value chain', which obviously would break when funding was over.

This is only one example of many (in particular mobile telephone) projects, representing vertical projects that are taking over and controlling subsets of data collection, particularly in Africa. An additional problem with the end-to-end model of cloud-based big data management was that the MoH had to pay for their own data. In Rwanda, an end-to-end provider established a system for the collection of disease surveillance data. The model of not owning your own data and having to pay for it was the reason why the system was closed down, and the data collection and management moved to the national routine HIS system.

The cloud-based service models and the use of mobile phones make it easy to establish systems and pilots with a limited scope. From the complexity model described, it is difficult to outsource systems with multiple interdependencies and components. Limited single purpose systems, such as the Vodafone system in the Gambia, on the other hand, are easy to outsource as services. The individual components in a complex system, which are delinked from the rest of the system, are not by themselves complex. But such delinking and removal from the national HIS, as in the Gambia, is a destructive way to create fragmentation while increasing the overall complexity.

At one point there were so many mobile projects in Uganda that the MoH intervened and made it mandatory to both get prior permission to start a project and to integrate their data with the national HIS data warehouse.

7.4.4 Complexity: Can health data and systems be black-boxed in service models?

Given the high level of complexity of contemporary ICT and information systems, the different service models described here are seen as a way for businesses to outsource the handling of complexity to service providers. Development of the cloud and big data may be seen as a transition of increasing sophistication through the various service models: Infrastucture, Platform, Software, and Analytics.

Based on the inherent openness and fuzziness of public health data and systems, some of their various components cannot go through such a transition of commodification and black-boxing. Efforts to achieve such commodification are important parts of the currently ongoing 'big data' and outsourcing efforts. An important question will be how such efforts to streamline everything as 'easy to go' boxes may eventually backfire and trigger the reopening of the black boxes and debunk beliefs of steady technological progress. This may then cause setbacks and the 'opening of the black boxes', or calling the bluff, if the plan has been to be the technology optimist. Such examples abound. Reverse salient is an old military research term, used by Thomas Hughes (1983) on setbacks in infrastructure development when it has been too fast or too poorly grounded. In military terms, reverse salient is when one part of the frontline becomes weak and the enemy threatens to break through, and the whole frontline has to step back and consolidate.

The example of the DHIS 2 implementation in a big African country where the metadata structure had been developed ad hoc, is a good illustration of a reverse salient. While the system was in the process of being rolled out after a pilot period, performance of the system deteriorated as more provinces and users were added. Poor metadata design caused the server to crash when many users logged in. This revelation came only one and a half years into the process, representing a breakdown and the opening of the black box in the Thomas Hughes sense. Poorly designed systems will ultimately break down. The health information exchanges and use areas supported and encompassed by the HIS in a typical country-level HMIS implementation are highly context-sensitive and complex, with many linkages to different organizational structures and 'moving' parts. We have seen that the DHIS 2 platform is gaining tremendous popularity, but this in itself can push it into getting black-boxed. Huge potential of breakdowns will be created if designs are not sensitive to the health system complexities and are not allowed the time and space to adapt, evolve, and embed themselves in new contexts.

On another note, the history of DHIS versions 1 and 2 until now may be analysed in the light of reverse salient, where performance of certain components of the dominant—and always very techno-optimist—paradigm fails. Until now, DHIS 2 has had the role of the tortoise in Aesop's fable about the tortoise and the hare, while larger technology projects have taken the role of the hare. DHIS has always been slowly walking forward regardless of the current fashion. In this new situation of increasing international donor acceptance of DHIS 2 and the rapid expansion and increased complexity in each country, DHIS 2 may risk taking over the role of the hare!

7.4.5 Concluding remarks on black-boxing services and big data

In the discussion in section 7.4.4 we have concluded that HIS and big health data cannot be commodified, black-boxed, and outsourced to service providers. This highlights the importance of the veracity dimension of big data.

However, the possible messiness and poor quality of health data are consequences of this complexity. Complexity is the root cause for why health data and HIS cannot be black-boxed, and need to be included in our understanding of big data. International hosting will typically provide a far better techno-commercial option than local hosting. Governments, however, want to store their data within the country's borders, not in the unspecified cloud. For the development of HIS, it is important to aim at leveraging all the advantages of cloud-based computing, while ensuring that the risks are well mitigated and managed. This is a non-trivial task given the institutional work required.

7.5 Approaches to Handling Complexity in Public Health Information Systems in Low and Middle-Income Countries

In this last section, we summarized the key issues related to complexity and how the Expanded PHI approach can help to design strategies to manage HIS complexity in LMIC contexts.

We have argued that the context of public health in LMICs is characterized by being less formalized and structured than, say, in hospitals in industrialized countries. The concept of outreach services in public health is in contrast to the more formalized 'inward' reaching services carried out within the walls of a hospital. Outreach activities aiming at, for example, providing services to children and mothers that are not reached by the facility-based health services illustrates the openness in terms of the scope of data collection and systems, the linkages to society, and context of use in population-based systems.

In the model presented, complexity is seen to increase with context sensitivity and number of connections or interdependencies with other systems. We have discussed several concepts used to understand how higher levels of complexity influence HIS development and data quality: poorly formalized business procedures; fuzziness of data; a web of connections to the social system; open-endedness in terms of the scope of the system; and higher levels of context sensitivity. In system development, these aspects of complexity may be translated into levels of uncertainty related to the context and goals of the system to be developed, as well as to the system development process as such.

Systems development, whether it is about strengthening existing systems or developing a new one, such as the integrated solution in Indonesia, is, at a basic level, about identifying what needs to be done and then doing it, or to define tasks, and then carrying them out. The less complex the situation, the more the system can be predefined, and more of the development can be properly planned and defined before it is actually carried out. The opposite is also true—the more complexity and higher the level of uncertainty, the less development can be planned in advance. Of course, roadmaps and general directions of work can always be prepared, but the concrete medium to longer-term plans will need to be developed and revised as part of the building process.

When uncertainty related to the context and goals of system development is high, experimental approaches, user participation and learning by doing are generally recommended (Andersen *et al.* 1986; Davis 1982). These are approaches within the concept of cultivation. When the uncertainty is high, development may not be controlled totally, but a cultivation strategy which incorporates user participation, tinkering, improvisation, and gradual development over time is an important approach to managing uncertainty. Attractors may be sought, created as a strategy to guide the direction of design and development. This cultivation approach may be seen as having two main components:

i) User participation, experiments around practical prototypes, and shared learning by doing among users and developers as part of the day-to-day development. Seek to develop and strengthen attractors for change through prototyping activities.

ii) An evolutionary and process-oriented approach. Accepting that development will take time and that piecemeal development and learning are needed to help guide further work.

Robust, flexible, and scalable system architectures are essential for systems development in contexts of high complexity and uncertainty, as it must always be possible to add components. It is therefore important to delay decisions that can close future choices as much as possible. During the first phase of developing the national system in South Africa during 1997–2000, user participation in the hands-on development of prototypes was an important part of the strategy (Braa and Hedberg 2002), involving iterative and continuous interactions between developers and users. This contributed to mutual learning where users learn to what extent and how their information needs could be implemented using the technology, and the developers learn about the context of use and users' needs. By default, the development of the national HIS in South Africa witnessed an evolutionary step-by-step approach as new modules and subsystems were included.

Also in the early phases of the process of the Indonesia project, practical prototypes for demonstrating what can be done with integrated data have been an important part of the interaction with the multitude of user groups and health programmes. Working towards integrated solutions in the highly complex context of Indonesia will need to be gradual and with a long-time horizon. In Ghana, we have seen that the process of strengthening the system and improving data quality has been carried out as an inclusive data review process, starting at the facility and district levels before moving to the regional and national levels. This process has resulted in improved data quality, which again has convinced other programmes and stakeholders, such as TB and HIV/AIDS, to join the process. All these examples are about cultivating an evolutionary process of system development, and also showing that attractors for change can help create a momentum for change. In Ghana, the attractor was the DHIMS 2 system, which has already achieved results in strengthening data quality.

Similarly, the data warehouse and dashboard have served as other effective attractors for change, and have helped to navigate through high degrees of complexity. Integrated statistical data warehouse and dashboard systems have been relatively successful because they are not closely embedded in complicated business processes, and can stand 'above' it. Furthermore, they have a flexible and scalable architecture, allowing for adding new data sets and components as needs arise and new actors join. Such scalability would not have been possible at a general level in the context of more complicated business models. Data input and outputs are relatively simple processes and are not restricted to any place in a particular business process. The dashboard is loaded with data behind the scene; the user can access the data through the internet, from any physical position, and, particularly in this context, from any place or stage in any business or work process. Of course, the data being presented may be more or less useful, but to design useful dashboards for different user groups is relatively easy. Data collection is more complex, but provided resources, it is achievable. In cases similar to Indonesia, where a lot of existing data sources are electronic, collaboration and agreements between system owners and other stakeholders are the keys to success. Technically, it is relatively easy to import data into a data warehouse installed on a central server. Paper-based data collection and data sources, however, have their own complexities and problems related to data quality, which are not solved by a system on a central server. But the procedures for collecting routine data from health facilities have been established over many years in most countries and are fairly formalized, and easy to computerize.

Our Expanded PHI approach emphasizes the need for modern technologies, such as the use of central servers for cloud computing, sensitively coupled with thoughtful design and development approaches that understand and factor in the complexity that characterizes this domain.

7.6 **References**

Adaletey, D., Jolliffe, B., Braa, J., Ofosu, A. (2014). Peer-performance review as a strategy for strengthening health information systems: A case study from Ghana. *Journal of Health Informatics in Africa*, 2(2).

Andersen, N.E., Kensing, F., Lundin, J., *et al.* (1986). *Professional System Development.* Teknisk Forlag, Copenhagen, Denmark.

Berg, M. (1997). Of forms, containers, and the electronic medical record: some tools for a sociology of the formal. *Science, Technology and Human Values,* **22**(4), 403–33.

Braa, J., Hanseth, O., Mohammed, W., Heywood, A., Shaw, V. (2007). Developing health information systems in developing countries: The flexible standards approach. MIS Quarterly, **31**(2), 381–402.

Braa, J. and **Hedberg, C.** (2002). The struggle for district based health information systems in South Africa. *The Information Society,* **18**, 113–27.

Ciborra, C.U. (1997). De profundis? Deconstructing the concept of strategic alignment. *Scandinavian Journal of Information Systems,* **9**(1), 67–82.

Dahlbom, B. and **Janlert, J.E.** (1996). *Computer Future (manuscript).* Dept. of Informatics, Gothenburg University, Sweden.

Davis G.B. (1982). Strategies for information requirements. *IBM System Journal,* **21**, 4–30.

Eoyang, G. (1996). Complex? Yes! Adaptive? Well, maybe… *Interactions,* **3**(1), 31–7.

Foucault, M. (1975). *The Birth of the Clinic,* Vintage Books, New York, NY.

Galtung J. (1971). Structural theory of imperialism. *Journal of Peace Research,* **8**(2), 81–117.

Greenbaum, J. (1998). From Chaplin to Dilbert: the origins of computer concepts. In: **Arrowitz, S.** and **Culter, J.** (eds.). *Post-work.* Routledge, New York, NY.

Hughes, T. (1983) *Networks of Power: Electrification in Western Society, 1880–1930.* Johns Hopkins University Press, Baltimore, MD.

Jervell, H.R. (1991). Artificial intelligence and artificial environments. In: **Rønning, I.H.** and **Lundby, K.** (eds.) Media and communication. *Readings in Methodology, History and Culture,* pp. 169–77. Universitetsforlaget, Oslo, Norway.

Kirkebøen, G. (1993). *Psychology, Information Technology, and Expertise. A study of the impact of information technology in psychology—and vice versa.* Institute for Linguistics and Philosophy, University of Oslo, Norway (in Norwegian).

Kling, R. and **Scacchi, W.** (1982). The web of computing: Computer technology as social organisation. *Advances in Computers,* **21**, 1–90.

Laney, D. (2001). *3-D Data Management: Controlling Data Volume, Velocity and Variety.* META Group Original Research Note.

Plsek, P.E. and **Wilson, T.** (2001). Complexity science: Complexity, leadership, and management in healthcare organisations. *British Medical Journal,* **323**(7315), 746–9.

Poppe, O., Jolliffe, B., Adaletey, D., Braa, J., Manya, A. (2013). Cloud computing for health information in Africa? Comparing the case of Ghana to Kenya. *Journal of Health Informatics in Africa,* **1**(1).

Popper, K. ([1957], 1986). *The Poverty of Historicism,* Routledge, London, UK.

Rodrigues, R.J. and **Israel, K.** (1995). *District-based Information Systems.* Pan American Health Organization/WHO.

Stephen, S., Lim, S.S., Stein, D.B., Charrow, A., Murray, C. (2008). Tracking progress towards universal childhood immunisation and the impact of global initiatives: a systematic analysis of three-dose diphtheria, tetanus, and pertussis immunisation coverage. *The Lancet,* **372**(9655), 2031–46.

Chapter 8

Measuring Progress Towards Universal Health Coverage and Post-2015 Sustainable Development Goals: The Informational Challenges

8.1 Introduction: Scope of Contemporary Informational Challenges

Expectations from health information systems (HIS) in low and middle-class countries (LMICs) have risen considerably in recent times, contributed to by the coming centre-stage of the universal health coverage (UHC) discourse and the related push to strengthen the civil registration and vital statistics (CRVS) systems. Interlinked to this is the emphasis on the post-2015 Sustainable Development Goals (SDGs) which replaced the Millennium Development Goals (MDGs) in 2015. The requirement of 'measurement of progress towards the SDGs' contributes to expanding the scope and quality of public health informatics support required.

This chapter covers three themes. The first theme concerns the key problems of measuring progress towards UHC and the post-2015 SDGs, and their implications on the required supporting information. We also discuss the current initiative on the Health Data Collaborative, which explicitly seeks to strengthen the supporting HIS. The second theme discusses each of the four data sources—population surveys, primary care service data, hospital information, and CRVS—and how they each need to be rethought and restructured in order to meet the emerging needs. The third and final theme emphasizes the need to align these four data sources with one another, guided by the framework architecture of Expanded PHIs. But architecture is itself a problematic—with different ideologies and contexts shaping it in varied, often contradictory ways. It is only an expanded understanding of PHI that could help address these complexities.

8.2 Understanding Universal Health Coverage: Implications for Information Support

8.2.1 Origins and definition

The current emphasis on UHC gained prominence after the 2005 World Health Organization Assembly resolution (WHO 2005), which called for nations to work towards universal coverage, and the subsequent World Health Report of 2008—'Primary Healthcare—Now More Than Ever' (World Health Report 2008)—carried a chapter devoted to UHC. Subsequently, a considerable number of papers have further developed this concept, including the WHO's World Health Report 2010, which exclusively elaborated the theme of health systems financing around UHC. Various nations have set up commissions or expert groups to recommend strategies on how to progress towards UHC. In 2012, the United Nations adopted a resolution declaring UHC as the goal for all health systems[i], and the World Bank and Rockefeller Foundation initiated a series of publications in the form of country-specific case studies on UHC.

The WHO 2010 report defined UHC as 'the desired outcome of health system performance whereby all people who need health services (promotion, prevention, treatment, rehabilitation and palliation) receive them, without undue financial hardship' (WHO 2010). This is similar to the idea of affordable, accessible healthcare for all that the earlier discourse of 'Health for All by 2000 AD'. had emphasized.

A key change is the emphasis on measurement of service coverage and financial risk protection coverage. This mainstreaming of measurement highlights the need for high-level informatics support, which however has not been a topic of discussion around the current UHC discourses (Sahay *et al.* 2015).

8.2.2 Current discourses on universal health coverage in the global health community and its relation to providing information support

The challenge of achieving equity within UHC is regarded as the major challenge in the ongoing discourse on UHC in the global health community. To develop approaches to measure various aspects of coverage are representing the informational challenges linked to the quest for equity. The first level of measuring equity within UHC is related to who is getting included and who is getting excluded from the various health services, and from the supporting insurance schemes. In a literature review of research on equity within UHC, Rodney and Hill (2014), concludes that there is a changing position of equity within the UHC agenda in current research from 'being viewed as an integral component and implied outcome of UHC, to more recently being seen as a complex but measurable indicator of UHC success'. (*ibid.*, p. 6). This recent contextualization of UHC has led to the development of tools, frameworks, and indicators to better measure equity within UHC. An interesting finding from the reviewed research was that UHC programmes should first of all focus on increasing coverage among the most disadvantaged groups, as this approach will lead to increased coverage in all income groups. In cases where such a pro-poor approach were not followed, uptake in the overall population seemed to be slower. This finding may be seen as a confirmation of Gwatkin and Ergo's (2011) quest for affirmative action to reach the poor, an approach they labelled 'progressive universalism'. They aimed at changing the trend of trickle-down patterns in countries implementing UHC, where new health programmes first tended to reach the higher income groups before, gradually—if at all—then trickle down to disadvantaged groups. Rather, they suggested that health programmes should target the poor first and ensure that they gain at least as much as those who are better off, rather than having to wait and catch up later. The importance of ensuring that the poor have access to more comprehensive health care packages and not limited to a chosen few highly selective incentives has also been emphasized.

Another interesting finding in Rodney and Hill's (2014) review of research on equity in UHC is a warning that the current insurance model in many LMICs is not to promote public provision of high-demand primary care, but the privatization of more profitable tertiary services. This trend, they argue, is weakening the already fragile public health systems and will therefore increase inequity by decreasing the efficiency of the publicly funded health system. On this background, they conclude that achieving equity within UHC requires a holistic approach focused on accessible and high quality primary, secondary and tertiary healthcare (*ibid.*).

Lessons we can draw from the above arguments on approaches to provide information support to UHC are, first, that the approaches advocated in this book of focusing on disadvantaged groups and measuring coverage of health services for them are still of key importance. However, second, as the traditional approach towards disadvantaged groups tends to focus on few primary healthcare services, we need to extend our approach to include coverage among disadvantaged groups also of a more comprehensive primary care package, as well as of secondary and tertiary healthcare. As the traditional approaches of measuring coverage of disadvantaged groups tend to be linked to health services at locations and geography, where denominators can be identified, these approaches need to be expanded by additional ways to measure coverage of secondary and tertiary services in disadvantaged groups by other means (e.g. such as through surveys), and to integrate with data from hospital information systems.

Another challenge related to equity within UHC in LMICs is related to the way the health insurance schemes are designed and implemented. The problem is that the poor and people from the informal sector are not easily reached by more or less voluntary health insurance schemes, which are based on people pre-paying for coverage, and together pool the risks. This is the reason why the 'trickle down' approach referred to above, where the well-off and people from the formal sector are being reached first, by default, remains the trend for how health insurance is implemented in LMICs. The case of Ghana is illustrative: Ghana has implemented a National Health Insurance Scheme since 2004 based on a model of contribution, with some groups exempted from contributing. How to fund people from the informal sector has been debated: should it be paid through tax, or through a particular system of individual contribution as a one-time premium (Abiiro and McIntyre 2012). This debate of pro et contra public funding for the poor and those in the informal sector has not yet yielded results, as the following summary of the situation in Ghana from Nyonator *et al.* (2014) reveals: 'NHIS coverage in 2012 was 34% of the population compared to the target of 70%. Designed to be pro-poor, membership on NHIS favours the middle-wealth quintiles. Out-of-pocket health expenditure remained the same at just under 30% of total health expenditure'. (Nyonator *et al.* 2014)

There are numerous recommendations for LMICs to replace private voluntary financing with compulsory public systems where employers and employees covers formal sector and use mostly tax financing to cover informal sectors. In addition to the general problem of reaching the poor, membership-based insurance schemes in LMICs tend also to have a problem with people stuck in the middle, who are too poor to pay for insurance, but not poor enough for being supported by government and NGO-administered schemes.

The 'universal' in UHC is defined as an obligation by the state to provide healthcare to all its citizens, but as noted by O'Connell *et al.* (2014), many groups are falling outside this obligation and the term 'universal' is applied differently across countries. Either deliberately or passively, many countries are not providing adequate health services to particular groups, be they stateless, unregistered, nomads, refugees, or slum dwellers in big cities. Migrant workers, refugees, and other population groups not formally registered represent an informational challenge, and a challenge in reaching full coverage. For example, in China, the internal migrant population exceeded 250 millons in 2012. Of this population, 160 million were without household registration, the 'floating population', and therefore regarded as aliens in their own nation and only with difficulty reached by the public health services (Armstrong 2012). Kuwait is solving their 'problem' of having defined about 100,000 people living within their borders as stateless people, by offering them citizenship in the Comores

Island in a deal with that country. The refugee exodus from Syria and its neighbouring countries and the crisis in Europe is another example of the challenges of making the UHC really universal; for all people regardless of their status. It is (also) an informational challenge to provide adequate health services to the population groups referred to here, but it is first of all a political problem of granting them the right to services.

Comparing data from the regular health management information systems (HMIS) with the insurance systems, or simply registering those without membership, will show the proportion of groups falling outside the health insurance schemes. Categorization of the client as refugee, stateless, etc. may help the measuring of what extent these groups are being reached. The issue of a client to the health services either being a member or not being a member in the insurance scheme is an important informational aspect when providing supporting to UHC. While the traditional HMIS which may or may not record all clients and all services provided in a facility, the insurance system based on EMRs will only record members of the insurance scheme and services eligible for refunding. Appropriate integration of these two types of systems and comparison of the two types of data are important in measuring coverage of the UHC, and it may be used to identify population groups with poor coverage.

8.2.3 **Measurement of universal health coverage**

A small cube nested within a larger one, as shown in Figure 8.1, usually depicts the scope of measurement for UHC. The breadth of the larger cube represents

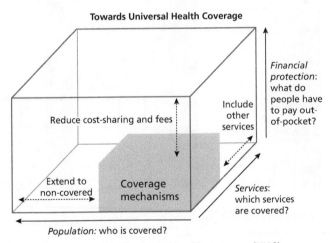

Fig. 8.1 Scope of measurement of universal health coverage (UHC).

Reproduced with permission from WHO, *Health financing for universal coverage: Universal coverage—three dimensions*, http://www.who.int/health_financing/strategy/dimensions/en/, accessed 01 Feb. 2016, Copyright © 2016 WHO.

the population to be covered by a service, and the breadth of the smaller cube within is the proportion of population currently effectively covered by the service. The depth of the larger cube would be ideally the entire range of quality health services required by that population, and that of the smaller cube is the priority services that are currently available. The height of the larger cube is total cost of the services, and the smaller cube represents the proportion of costs met by financial protection mechanisms, such as government subsidies or insurance. In this depiction, the ideal is the large outer cube, while the inner cube represents current reality, and the movement from the inner to the outer cube along each axis measures progress towards UHC (Boerma *et al.* 2014).

This depiction of progress may be deceptively simple, but in practice this measurement is complex and problematic and must satisfy two purposes (Sahay and Sundararaman 2015). One of these is to make summary assessment of the status of a nation, which finds use in cross-country comparisons and provides impetus for policy interventions to maintain or improve performance.

Most such approaches use a subset of tracer indicators for measuring coverage, and combine it with financial protection indicators available from periodic surveys; either into a single index, or a set of indicators (see Fig. 8.2). Most LMICs do not have an adequate database to calculate these coverage indicators,

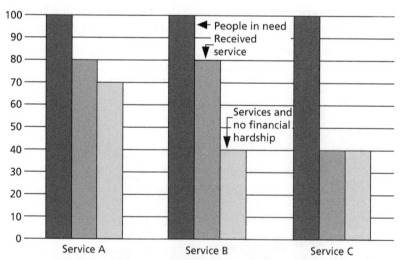

Fig. 8.2 Proposed indicators for measuring progress towards UHC.

and tend to continue to rely on the existing MDG database. Even with limited indicators, reliability is a problem.

The other purpose of measurement is to enable public health management action at subnational levels. In large nations like India, such action is primarily the responsibility of the provincial or state level, with the federal government having a role in financing and in redressing uneven development. Provincial governments require health sector performance metrics—disaggregated by districts and below—to identify those lagging behind, and provision to fill the financial, human, and knowledge-related gaps. In addition, governments need to decide priority services to be included in an insurance package or made available as assured services, and the mechanisms by which to ensure financial protection. And for all of this, accurate information is required on what services people require most, which services contribute most to costs of care, patterns of service utilization, and effective models of financial protection. It is not essential that both these purposes be served by the same approach to measurement. Survey-based approaches, which are time and cost intensive, would be useful to generate national UHC progress scores on select indicators. Measuring progress towards UHC using routine data will provide more granular and relevant information to guide policy and management choices, but would require the existing systems to be improved and expanded considerably.

With this understanding of measurement, in the next section we examine some challenges before any HIS.

8.2.4 **Health informatics-related challenges**

Measuring service coverage on the x-axis

The information required is 'the proportion of persons in need of a particular service who were able to access that service in a given time period'. Almost all nations currently measure coverage for immunization, antenatal care services, or services of a skilled birth attendant. The indicators would be:

- Percentage of all children below one year of age in a district who were fully immunized.
- Percentage of all pregnant women in the last one year who received the full package of four antenatal check-ups.
- Percentage of deliveries attended to by a skilled birth attendant.

If the local health facility has a nurse providing antenatal care services, we cannot conclude that all pregnant women living in the catchment area of that facility are covered. Other than physical access, there are financial, social, or behavioural barriers to overcome. We also do not measure the declaration of an entitlement as coverage. If delivery services are included as a part of the insurance programme in which pregnant women are enrolled, that would not be considered as coverage. We would insist on counting only those women who received these services—the term used being 'effective coverage'. Effective coverage represents the fraction of potential health gain actually delivered to the population through the health system as based on the three components of NEED, USE, and QUALITY. NEED refers to the individual/population in need of a particular service; USE refers to the use of services; and QUALITY refers to the actual health benefit experienced (Ng *et al.* 2014). While effective coverage is important, as it allows for a much better measure of progress towards universal coverage, it is complex, as it needs to be done for each service separately and it needs to factor in quality.

In the context of LMICs, extending the metrics beyond preventive reproductive and child healthcare poses a number of challenges (Sundararaman *et al.* 2014). Let us take the example of hypertension. In a UHC scenario, in a given district, every adult would be screened for hypertension and those detected as having hypertension would, after a physician consultation, be put on a therapeutic regime with periodic follow-up visits which the primary care provider can guide. In the event of developing complications they would be referred for specialist consultation at the district hospital, following which the primary care provider will provide the follow-up. The primary health centre would be able to provide the following indicators:

i)   incidence rate of new hypertension cases
ii) hypertension prevalence rate
iii) percentage of hypertensives who are regular in attending check-ups
iv) percentage of hypertensives whose blood pressure is well controlled
v)   incidence rate of complications
vi) hypertension or cardiovascular disease related mortality rates.

This is not an impossible or unrealistic task, and is effectively undertaken in high-income nations built around a strong primary care approach. In the United Kingdom, the National Health Service not only measures it, but also provides monetary incentives to primary care physicians who do well in maintaining blood pressure in the normal range for all hypertensives in their service area. Among LMICs, Thailand and Brazil have primary care systems that provide this extent and quality of coverage.

However, most LMICs would have problems in generating the above indicators. Hypertension prevalence rate, a measure of NEED for services, is difficult to obtain in the absence of a systematic programme for annual blood pressure check-up and recording for all adults. If check-up visits are random and not fixed to particular providers, it is highly likely to have unrecorded or duplicated cases. Part of the duplication problem could be attributed to the lack of use of unique identifiers, which technically could be relatively easy to solve, but institutionally becomes problematic as the different providers and their systems would not communicate with one other, or use an uniform identifier. Many LMICs use the strategy of opportunistic screening, where every adult over 30 years of age who comes to a health facility for whatever reason is screened for blood pressure. This would fail to detect hypertension in asymptomatic patients who do not come to any facility, plus lead to double counting of those patients visiting multiple facilities. Thus, measuring the USE of services by known patients is also a challenge. There is no one provider or facility responsible for the control of hypertension. As a result, this aggregate data of proportion of service users whose blood pressure was controlled—which would represent a population-based estimate of QUALITY of care—is just not collected or computed. Measuring disease-specific mortality and morbidity rates is also a challenge.

If this is the challenge with just one disease—hypertension—measuring this for *all* diseases is a challenge multiplied manifold. For many other diseases arriving at the 'population in need of services' would be an even greater challenge, as would also the measures of use and quality of care. Some high-income nations derive these statistics from disease-based registries, such as the Scandinavian nations, or from primary care networks which have universal coverage, like the United Kingdom. But in the absence of such systems, even rich countries will have problems in generating population-based statistics.

For communicable diseases like tuberculosis, HIV, leprosy, and vector-borne diseases, most LMICs have established reasonably functional and robust disease surveillance systems to help measure NEED in terms of incidence and prevalence of the disease, USE based on number of patients placed on treatment, and QUALITY in terms of effectiveness of care measured by reduction in morbidity and mortality in those on treatment. However this sort of surveillance, use, and outcome data is unavailable for measuring most diseases. In India, for example, communicable diseases that come under national communicable disease programmes account for less than 6 per cent of all morbidities and less than 20 per cent of morbidities due to communicable diseases. Measuring coverage for other communicable diseases therefore remains a challenge.

This measurement of effective coverage can be made for each disease and the number of diseases theoretically measured in the z-axis, which represents the size of the assured package of financially protected services. One option is to do away with the z-axis and present progress towards UHC separately for each category of services as a series of two-dimensional bar charts. Another is to commit to a global normative set of, say, 100 essential services, and measure what proportion of these a nation has been able to include in its essential package. A third, and perhaps the most misleading option, is to measure whatever services the nation has currently committed to—typically a small package of reproductive and child health services and two or three national disease control programmes. This approach is often taken in a number of studies, but runs against the spirit and expectations of UHC.

Measuring financial protection on the y-axis

The nature of the problem in measuring on the y-axis is entirely different. Unlike with coverage, commonly used metrics for financial protection do not measure the height of the small cube representing what is protected. Rather, they measure the gap—*the lack* of financial protection—as different from *the extent* of financial protection. In many situations, the covered costs representing the extent of financial protection are unknown. This creates considerable problems in calculating the proportion of total health expenditure that is protected. The common measures for *lack* of financial protection are:

i) Out-of-pocket expenditure (OOPE) per person per year: Closely related measures are OOPE per hospitalization episode and service specific OOPEs, such as for normal delivery services, or for one month's ambulatory care for diabetes. These could be averaged to OOPE per outpatient visit or per inpatient episode, presented as both the mean and the median.

ii) Incidence of catastrophic health expenditures (CHE): This is the proportion of *households* in a population that face CHE, representing instances when the healthcare costs exceed 10 (or 25) per cent of the total household expenditures, or 20 (or 40) per cent of the non-food expenditure. The implication is that at this level of expenditure, other essential expenses of the family are compromised. Such information—typically collected through household surveys which measure total annual household expenditure on food, on non-food items, and on healthcare separately in order to compute proportions per 100 households that had experienced CHE in the previous year—is the measure of financial hardship.

iii) Mean positive catastrophic health expenditure overshoot: Percentage points by which household spending on health exceeds the threshold for catastrophic health expenditure. This is a relatively less used indicator. Whereas the earlier indicator is based on a yes/no measure of CHE, this indicator provides an estimate of the extent of financial hardship.

iv) Incidence of impoverishment due to health expenditure: This is the number of households in which the net household expenditure computed after removing healthcare costs falls below the poverty threshold measure used to define poverty in that nation. Net household expenditure is the total consumption expenditure of the household minus the health expenditure. This is useful to measure the financial hardship caused in nations where a large part of the population lives close to poverty. Of course this indicator would fail to count those already in poverty, who became even more impoverished.

v) Increase in extent of poverty: This is the amount by which a household fell further into poverty due to health spending.

All these are measures of the lack of financial protection. Distinct from these, in most LMICs, the computation of the extent of financial protection requires an estimation of total health expenditure where public health expenditure and insurance payments, and direct employer payments are factored in. Non-OOPE expenditures, as a proportion of total health expenditure, provide an estimate of financial protection. Even in contexts where all payments to providers are presumably from insurance, it is important to measure out-of-pocket expenditure as well as public expenditure, since either or both of these could be substantial. Nominal financial protection in the form of enrolment in an insurance scheme could vary widely from effective financial protection in terms of experiencing cashless services when in need.

Such an approach to estimating financial protection—public health expenditures plus pre-payment as a percentage of total health expenditures—is a useful indicator for comparing performance in financial protection across nations. However since there are considerable inefficiencies in public expenditure and in insurance-financed care, the quantum of public health expenditure does not reflect the level of financial protection it provides. Similarly, there is the possibility of considerable overconsumption of care in the private sector, and a considerable part of OOPE may be unnecessary or optional—such as better quality of private wards or boutique delivery care. In Brazil, for example, public health expenditure represents about 50 per cent of total health expenditure, but over 70 per cent of all healthcare provision. In India public health expenditure represents about 29 per cent of total health expenditure but about 33 per cent of healthcare provision (excluding unqualified providers), about 40 per cent of inpatient care, and almost all preventive and promotive public health services.

Thus for purposes of policy, planning, and guiding implementation, it is the 'lack of financial protection' measured as OOPE and the incidence of CHE that is currently used. Again, while it may be possible to make a combined index of lack of financial protection, most sources would prefer to have a dashboard where all four or five indicators of OOPE and their impact on the household is displayed. Other useful indicators include percentage of those who are covered by an insurance scheme, or percentage of outpatient and inpatient care that occurs in tax-funded public health facilities providing free or subsidized care.

8.3 **Measuring the Post-2015 Sustainable Development Goals**

The post-2015 SDGs show many points of convergence with the UHC agenda, but also some clear differences. The post-2015 agenda as adopted in the UN special session in September 2015 has 9 aims and 17 goals. Of the 17 SDGs, only one is directly dedicated to health, which states 'Ensure healthy lives and promote well-being for all at all ages'. This goes beyond maternal and child survival and vertical disease control programmes that characterized the MDGs. However, all the health-related MDGs remain in the SDG list, although now 'reduced' to sub-goals or targets as they are named. In addition, there are at least seven other SDGs that relate to key social determinants of health. The third SDG related to health has nine targets, each underlying a significant public health informatics challenge, and four more which are described as 'targets for means of implementation'. The eighth of these targets is to 'Achieve universal health coverage, including financial risk protection, access to quality essential healthcare services and access to safe, effective, quality, and affordable essential medicines and vaccines for all'. The nine targets related to health outcomes and outputs and the four related to means of implementation are presented in Table 8.1:

Table 8.1 Sustainable Development Goals: the nine sub-goals of Goal-3

Target 1	By 2030, reduce the global maternal mortality ratio to less than 70 per 100,000 live births
Target 2	By 2030, end preventable deaths of newborns and children under 5 years of age
Target 3	By 2030, end the epidemics of AIDS, tuberculosis, malaria, and neglected tropical diseases and combat hepatitis, water-borne diseases, and other communicable diseases
Target 4	By 2030, reduce by one-third premature mortality from non-communicable diseases through prevention and treatment, and promote mental health and well-being
Target 5	Strengthen the prevention and treatment of substance abuse, including narcotic drug abuse, and harmful use of alcohol
Target 6	By 2020, halve the number of global deaths and injuries from road traffic accidents
Target 7	By 2030, ensure universal access to sexual and reproductive healthcare services, including for family planning, information and education, and the integration of reproductive health into national strategies and programmes

Target 8	Achieve universal health coverage, including financial risk protection, access to quality essential healthcare services and access to safe, effective, quality, and affordable essential medicines and vaccines for all
Target 9	By 2030, substantially reduce the number of deaths and illnesses from hazardous chemicals and air, water, and soil production and contamination
Targets	**Targets for means of implementation:**
a	Strengthen the implementation of the World Health Organization Framework Convention on Tobacco Control in all countries, as appropriate
b	Support the research and development of vaccines and medicines for the communicable and non-communicable diseases that primarily affect developing countries, provide access to affordable essential medicines and vaccines, in accordance with the Doha Declaration on the TRIPS Agreement and Public Health, which affirms the right of developing countries to use to the full the provisions in the Agreement on Trade-Related Aspects of Intellectual Property Rights regarding flexibilities to protect public health, and in particular, provide access to medicines for all
c	Substantially increase health financing and the recruitment, development, training, and retention of the health workforce in developing countries, especially in the least developed countries and small island developing states
d	Strengthen the capacity of all countries, in particular developing countries, for early warning, risk reduction, and management of national and global health risks

As compared with the MDGs, the SDGs are vastly expanded across sectors including in all 169 targets. In fact, most of the critiques of the SDGs are claiming that the number of targets are too high: when you try to do everything, you end up achieving nothing. *The Economist* calls them the 169 commandments, and recommends them to follow Moses and prune them to 10 commandments: 'aimed squarely at reducing poverty, boosting education (for example, extending girls' schooling by two years) and improving health (say by halving the rate of malaria infection)' (The Economist 2015).

Previously we discussed some of the complexities of measuring UHC. But in the post-2015 list, that is only one of the nine sub-goals, and the other eight, which include with some modification all the health-related MDGs, are all challenging. Some common informational requirements emerge. First, lessons from measuring the MDGs, an important part of this book, remains valid; second is improved cause-of-death reporting, which requires more robust CRVS data. The third is improved inputs from disease surveillance systems for morbidity reporting. And fourth is improved quality of information from service delivery points of both primary and secondary care. And finally, there is the need for much better inter-sectoral reporting, such as finance, environmental pollution, transport, and others.

8.4 **Health Data Collaborative—International Partnership for Health Information and Tracking Health-related Sustainable Development Goals**

The Health Data Collaborative, launched by WHO and partner development agencies, countries, donors, and academics in March 2016, is a joint effort to work alongside countries to improve the quality of their health data and to track progress towards the health-related SDGs (http://www.who.int/features/2016/health-data-collaborative/en/; http://www.healthdatacollaborative.org/). This informal partnership of different actors explicitly aims to improve health data by strengthening country HIS, which can better support the emerging health reform initiatives.

The longer-term goals of the Health Data Collaborative is that by 2024, 60 LMICs, and supporting donors, will be using common investment plans to strengthen HIS, and that countries will not need international assistance for these systems by 2030. The practical approach is to establish a network of working groups that will address specific technical issues and a key part of this plan is to coordinate the various efforts to make sure everyone is pulling in the same direction. Through several working groups, the Health Data Collaborative will produce tools, templates, and data standards, such as required for public health management, hospital information systems, for disease surveillance, TB, malaria control, case-based investigation, and ICD10 mortality reporting.

The Health Data Collaborative is planning to become a strong global actor in the area of HIS, a bit similar to the Health Metrics Network exactly 10 years earlier, but with a different approach and organization. While HMN built a strong centralized organization and funded and organized projects to assess HIS and develop strategic plans in numerous countries, the Health Data Collaborative is focusing on a lean organization and on using a network of time-limited working groups as the main approach to operationalize activities. It sees itself as a facilitator bringing countries, donors, and other partners together to organize investments and is not intending to be responsible for financing HIS in countries.

8.5 **Data Sources**

8.5.1 **Existing situation**

The four major sources of data for UHC and SDGs are:

a) Household surveys: These are invaluable as they are the only means to measure a number of health events and associated costs as the community experiences it. They have two advantages: one, they capture events that occur in the private sector better; and two, they are relatively less influenced by the pressure on lower level managers to over-report service utilization and under-report adverse events.

b) Primary care provider data: This involves a record of health events with a reliable denominator—the population served by that primary care facility. It has problems of reliability since it is sourced as part of a disciplinary monitoring process. It also has considerable gaps in coverage, since much of the population is not clearly linked to a primary provider, and also because primary care practices tend to be highly selective, failing to take cognizance of most health events. The manual register-based system also poses challenges in monitoring coverage.

c) Facility-based medical care data: This is largely from hospitals, but would include curative care provided in mobile hospitals and clinics, which may not have inpatients. One potential source of such information is insurance claims data. Another source, more important in LMICs where effective insurance coverage is low, is data aggregated from hospital outpatient and inpatient records, typically done manually, with policy directions to move to electronic health records (EHRs).

d) Civil registration and vital statistics (CRVS): All nations have a registrar for births and deaths, and usually the same office is responsible for the census. Birth records plus census are key to estimating denominators of most coverage indicators. CRVS systems have yet to successfully address migrations and even to include marriages, and tend to be weak in death reporting, especially reliable causes of death. Almost all post-2015 SDGs' health sub-goals depend on these for burden of disease and cause of death estimates.

How can these data sources be made more relevant and reliable to meet the information needs of UHC and SDGs? An 'Expanded Public Health Informatics' is argued for, which aligns across these multiple data sources, representing what we call the architecture of public health informatics. This is now discussed in the next section.

8.5.2 Rethinking and restructuring data sources

Household surveys

While there are many different types of household surveys, those relevant to UHC and post-2015 agenda are discussed next.

i) Cost of care studies: Community-based sample surveys are essential because they collect data on total household consumption and incomes, in addition to data on morbidity and cost of healthcare. Though cost of care data can be recovered from insurance records, these would be serious under-estimates of out-of-pocket expenses, even among insured patients. In most LMICs, a majority of the population is not covered by insurance, or is covered on paper, but in practice not benefitting or often not even aware of it.

ii) Self-reported morbidity and access to care surveys: These are essential to uncover data on those who failed to access care or who accessed care from facilities not linked to the HMIS, typically the non-government ones. Self-reported morbidity under-reports a number of illnesses, partly because some of them are latent and not yet been diagnosed, and others because they are chronic and relatively uncomplicated, such as a hypertensive under care and on regular drugs. As a result, reported morbidity rates could vary widely across population groups based on what is perceived and reported as illness and on access and utilization of healthcare. Certain global protocols like SAGE (WHO Study on Global Ageing and Adult Health) have considerably reduced the problem by asking a well-planned set of queries instead of only one or two. There are many ways to limit problems of self-reported morbidity surveys, but none that overcomes them completely.

iii) Health examination surveys: These are household surveys where a clinician or trained paramedic carries out examination for certain illnesses, such as those related to malnutrition, anaemia, hypertension, diabetes, mental illness, and screening for common cancers—breast, cervix, and oral. Very few nations have integrated such surveys with other household surveys reported earlier, and these typically exist as standalone surveys which help to provide good understanding of disease prevalence, need for services and effectiveness of care received.

Information and communications technologies (ICTs) provide the potential to rethink and restructure the population-based surveys; for example, by enabling computer-assisted personal interviews with pre-loaded interview schedules (called computerized personal interview systems—CIPS), digital transmission of records to a central server, and computerized analysis, all of which can dramatically increase the ease and accuracy of surveys. While such tools have been already introduced for small-scale research projects, they need to be disseminated more widely, along with capacity building in the use of these tools. An increasing proportion of large surveys have now shifted to capturing data on handheld devices and transmitting them to central servers for immediate analysis. The effective use of this approach could make a huge difference to the collection and use of survey-based information, and the conducting of shorter quick local surveys and exit interviews, allowing for the capture of district and subdistrict level data disaggregates. These tools need to be strengthened with better techniques for data validation to enable collecting more precise information on morbidity patterns and costs of care for a much larger range of diseases—and faster than has been done so far.

In terms of HIS, integration of routine HMIS and survey data has a great potential, in that survey data can be used to validate the HMIS data reported from the health facilities and vice versa. While survey data will typically either not cover the whole country or not be granular and local enough, HMIS data are both local and countrywide. By correlating the two data sources, both levels of analysis will benefit; the validity of survey data at local level may be assessed through correlation with HMIS data, and the quality of HMIS data can be estimated for the part of the country covered by the survey. This correlation approach will, of course, depend on the two data sources collecting similar data.

Primary healthcare data

In the LMIC context, it is useful to distinguish between primary care provider data and other facility-based data, as the former contains data on the health of the population registered in a geographical space earmarked as the 'service area' for the particular facility. Most primary care systems require frontline workers to make regular house visits to all houses in their service area to provide essential preventive services listed within the package of care.

To do this systematically, primary care providers need to maintain registers, typically about 20 in number, to record various data on reproductive healthcare, immunization, disease control programmes, births and deaths, and various others. Where the services increase, so does the burden of recording data and consolidating it into monthly reports. Even more complex is to develop reports with data disaggregated by social groups for purposes of understanding health inequities. Many countries have made efforts to revise registers, but have not been effective in designing a register which allows effective information support for recording, tracking, and reporting data.

Digitization of primary healthcare registers has the potential to do this, provided it helps to reduce the burden of work of the peripheral care provider and enables the care s/he provides. Unfortunately, as discussed in earlier chapters, it often becomes a tool for imposing another layer of data-related work on the field nurse and becomes more of a tool of her surveillance, rather than of enabling and empowerment. More often than not, the functionalities required for analysing and generating population-based information at the peripheral level are weak or non-existent. Such digitization is, however, a necessary condition for achieving universal and comprehensive primary care, and will remain one of the essential strategies for achieving UHC. For UHC, there is a need to build a database of salient health facts for every household and individual, organized around units of primary care provision and capable of aggregation to levels of district, state, and national UHC.

Hospital-related data

Most healthcare facilities providing curative care would have a hospital information system or would need to acquire it promptly. In the context of UHC, the hospital information system needs to: provide reports on morbidity and mortality data; enable continuity of care between providers from primary, secondary and tertiary levels; and support purchasing of care by third parties, such as insurance companies. Each of these three requirements poses conceptual and operational challenges, which we discuss briefly next.

Reporting morbidity and mortality

Most policy recommendations call for the adoption of the International Classification of Diseases 10 (ICD10) and its recent upgrade to ICD11. While rarely is such a recommendation resisted by a LMIC's government, progress on this requirement is extremely slow or non-existent, as these ICD lists are far too long and beyond the capacity of most hospital care providers to implement. Problems relating to lack of diagnostic confirmation, especially for tissual studies or autopsies, and multiple providers come with different conclusions. Most hospital providers therefore ask to make shortlists, which are more convenient for them to try to map them onto the ICD. However, there is no semantic interoperability across such shortlists. WHO has tried to address this issue by identifying 270 to 300 ICD codes and their subgroups. The other challenge is around developing population-based statistics of morbidity and mortality, especially addressing the problem of deduplication to avoid the same health event being counted more than once. Unique identifiers help, but marginally, often becoming a distraction from attending to the main issues, which are more institutional. Another solution being explored is a central, shared personal record, but while theoretically feasible, it has been difficult to materialize in practice, and is extremely resource-intensive to implement.

Yet another relevant architecture is having *relevant* individual health information transmitted back from hospitals to the primary care provider, who then merges this with their database to compute aggregate population figures. Unique identifiers help, but so do patient profiles and referral linkages. Clearly this requires institutions to lay down rules regarding which information has to be reported, its frequency and quality, and to whom it has to be sent.

Enabling continuity of care

One important function of HIS is to enable continuity of care, which is shaped by the choice of architecture. The OpenHIE architecture discussed in Chapter 4 proposes a central EHR into which all providers must necessarily 'write'. But other nations have shown preference for limited centralization to an exchange centre, through which the records maintained with different providers could be accessed by patients. In this approach, both the primary care and hospital care providers maintain information in their respective formats, and make it available to providers on patients' request. This requires rules of both semantic and technical interoperability to be observed and enforced. As a routine, even without requests for full or partial access, a case summary of care provided at the referral level can always be transferred on request. This case summary would include all the information required for casting the indicators of effective coverage. In most LMICs, indicators of effective coverage, which are necessarily population based, are best assembled at the primary care provider level—rather than at the hospital level.

Supporting purchase of care

One key principle of a UHC roadmap is the separation of the provider and purchasing functions and the purchasing and payer functions. Providers could be public or private, networked or discrete standalone clinics, or primary, or tertiary care providers. Purchasers could be the government operating directly or through an autonomous body, or an insurance company to which government or the users themselves have made the payment. A purchaser is the agency which pays the provider, while the payer is the service user, commonly referred to as the patient. The payer could pay directly to the provider, or pay a premium to the insurance company or tax to the government, which is deducted from their wages. Payments made directly are out-of-pocket, most common in LMICs, are considered the most regressive and undesirable, where patients have limited information and power to negotiate the price. Also the rich and the poor pay the same amount for the same service, although the poor patient requires much more protection. In many rich nations, the government is the single payer, collecting revenues through direct taxes, where the rich would be paying more tax than the poor. The government then empanels various private providers who provide services to the population, and reimburses the provider for these services at a negotiated price. The patient pays nothing at the point of use, or a token copayment. The government may hire an insurance company to empanel private providers and purchase services on their behalf. Here, the payer and purchasing functions get separated.

In what is known as the Bismarckian system, the organization of care is similar, except that employers and employees also contribute to their respective insurance plans. In many LMICs, government facilities provide free, or highly subsidized services directly, making the government the payer, purchaser, and provider. This was typical of socialist governments in many LMICs, with the additional feature that private providers were either not allowed or discouraged. As public investments declined, the proportion of care provided by private sector has enlarged without a parallel growth of insurance. In the move towards UHC, three trends can be discerned in the nature of the provider–purchaser split. In Thailand, a different arm of the government undertakes the purchasing function. Providers of both primary and hospital care are mainly public providers, with a small number of private providers. Segregation of the purchasing function to a different arm of the government enables potentially a more flexible and responsive form of resource allocation. In Mexico, the trend is towards a transition to an insurance-based system, while in Brazil there is increasing reliance on insurance in secondary and tertiary care, while primary care is state-based provisioning. In many nations, we see a mix of these three trends.

Clearly ICT tools are much needed for managing the separation of provider and purchase functions. To make payments, purchasing agencies require authenticated and reliable information on the quality and quantity of care provided by healthcare facilities to individuals. The information needs would also include monitoring adherence to the standard treatment guidelines issued to guard against unnecessary diagnostics and therapeutics while safeguarding the provider from resorting to defensive medicine, which would increase the costs of care.

Civil registration and vital statistics

Age and disease-specific mortality rates are indicators of the overall health status or quality of life of a population. Yet for most LMICs, this data is very weak and there exist limited mechanisms to capture it. Even when deaths occur in hospitals, systems for medical certification of cause of deaths are weak. For deaths at home or in the community, the challenge of getting this data is far more complex for the informal care provider and the paramedic has limited medical knowledge. There is often a lack of clarity on who is responsible for certification and the disease codes within which this is done.

The WHO (2014) published features of a good CRVS as performing functions related to: (i) recording occurrence of vital events, births, and deaths, and associated characteristics; (ii) notification to the appropriate CRVS authorities and its entry into official public records; (iii) issuance of certificates of birth, death, and causes of death to family members and relevant authorities; (iv) compilation, analysis, and interpretation of vital statistics based on information generated through registration and certification; and (v) archiving of individual records for future use by individuals and as part of public records.

A good CRVS system would help in strengthening mortality reporting (maternal, neonatal, infant, under-5), which is the single most useful measure of health systems outcomes. Mature systems are able to present these mortality reports disaggregated by age, sex, social group, and geography. Indeed one global single indicator for the post-2015 SDG that was considered is preventable mortality before the age of 70 with guidelines on what constitutes as preventable death. This figure can also be generated only when there are age and disease-specific mortality tables available. Reporting and registration is a legally mandated function, and requires all private care providers to be included in the data collection network. A good CRVS system would help to maintain a dynamic household-level database, in terms of their choice/allocation of primary care provider, to help ensure that no individual is left out.

LMICs have been struggling to strengthen their CRVS systems but for various institutional reasons (Ahoobim *et al.* 2012) it has been difficult to build coordination across the departments of health, civil registration, statistical offices, and the community. In many nations, the health department is legally mandated to function as the civil registration authority, but this is not always the case, hence necessitating departmental coordination. Another key challenge is bringing about legal and regulatory changes needed to link CRVS improvements with national identity management systems. Securing cooperation from the communities is crucial, but often difficult to establish. Birth and death certification needs to be positioned in the community as an entitlement of citizenship, requiring examination of the structure of incentives for early and complete registration and penalties for late registration and non-compliance. It would require reaching out to community leaders, funeral authorities, religious leaders, grassroots organizations, especially of women, and enabling their capacities and infrastructure to provide these reports. A well-functioning CRVS system should be enabled to explicitly link with evidence-based health and development strategies by providing relevant statistical and M&E-related outputs to different divisions of the government.

For improving maternal, newborn, and child health-related events, registration facilities need to be positioned as close as possible to populated areas and within large hospitals and healthcare facilities as relevant. To build the confidence of health staff to report on child deaths, stillbirths, abortions, and deaths, complete confidentiality must be assured. For capturing stillbirths, abortions, and early neonatal deaths, we need good systems of recording and following up on every pregnancy until the pregnancy outcome is known and registered. LMICs need to establish a clear business process or standard operating procedures to ensure hassle-free and prompt delivery of the birth certificate. This process must define who has what role in each context, and what to do when there are deviations from the norm. Furthermore, systems can catch up by introducing fixed birth registration days—or children who are not registered, but visit the healthcare facility for other preventive or curative healthcare can be provided with registration and certification. The ICT systems must necessarily support interoperability and exchange of information between the CRVS system, the primary care provider, and those managing the population database for the local area. Addressing these challenges is a complex task that needs to be supported by effective formative research inputs to understand the context-specific barriers where registration is low (e.g. non-registration until a newborn's naming ceremony), and ways to address these barriers.

Improving death registration requires the establishment of clear standard operating procedures for certification in different contexts—the home where the informant is a relative or a paramedic; the hospital where the doctor is usually but not invariably available; the differences between certifying the fact of death and the cause of death when the latter is shrouded with different levels of uncertainty—and how this data is coded, shared, analysed, and presented while maintaining confidentiality. There needs to be a clear strategy on how to trace and list unrecorded deaths. There is also a need for widespread training of doctors in primary care facilities on medical certification of death based on ICD, including situations where the cause of death has to be defined retrospectively by verbal autopsy, or when only symptom-based reporting is possible.

Each of the issues discussed here can be strengthened greatly by appropriate ICT interventions. Some examples include:

◆ ICT tools for death reporting with cause of death: These need to be flexible enough to adapt to the limitations in providing details in different contexts. The causes of death, for example, could be categorized into suspected, presumptive or confirmed causes (as is done in disease surveillance reporting) and then analysed with this attribute factored in.

◆ ICT tools for disseminating and training on standards for cause of death: These require provision of support for cause-of-death reporting using verbal post-event inquiry mapped to ICD codes. Such training is required not only for doctors in hospital settings, but also for nurses and paramedics in primary care and community settings.

◆ ICT tools for transferring information on births and deaths to population registries maintained by both primary care providers and civil authorities at regional and national levels.

◆ ICT tools for enabling speedier birth and death certification, provided as an entitlement to households, and as feedback to the community to help in completing gaps in the records.

ICT tools are essential but not sufficient to overcome institutional and legal barriers, and those related to organizational capacity and political prioritization. Also, even if the tools are in place, they need to meet the technical and institutional requirements of interoperability.

While the institutional changes required may take time to implement on a nationwide scale, it would be quite feasible to implement these in a few sample districts immediately. Other than acting as a pilot and helping to build capacity and systems to undertake this task of CRVS reform, such districts would also act as sentinel sites, providing valuable public health information on age and disease-specific mortality and morbidity rates.

In some nations, including India and China, a sample registration survey has been introduced where a small sample of primary sampling units are fixed. Here routine death reporting is backed up by supervisors who check on the data and do a verbal autopsy to get more details of the cause of death and then record it. Three such three-yearly reports have been released in India. This approach, though a part of CRVS, is a mid-ground between surveys and CRVS, and the samples can be extended if ICT tools are judiciously applied.

8.6 **Aligning Information Flows: The Architecture Problematic**

The challenge is not only of aligning and converging of the data sources described above, but also of the different vertical health programmes, with each having its own supporting information system. There are also other information streams from other sectors, such as the police which is a very good information source of injuries and deaths due to road traffic accidents, assaults, and suicides. The early childhood care programmes can provide relevant data on child malnutrition, while the work and employment department should have data pertaining to occupational illness.

Discussions on architecture to address these challenges reflect two broad approaches, which we will now discuss.

8.6.1 **The centralized electronic health record approach**

This approach mandates a single EHR for every person on one national server, irrespective of the provider or service user, and for whichever disease. These EHRs must be reasonably standardized to be able to extract the necessary public health information in uniform formats. Most centralized EHR proposals envisage introduction of new software to which all systems and users will migrate—as if beginning with a clean slate. For example, the 12th Five Year Plan for India calls for 'A robust and effective HMIS which, in the best case scenario, tracks every health encounter and would enable assessment of performance and help in allocating resources to facilities'. Furthermore, India proposes a National eHealth Authority (NeHA) for the standardization, storage, and exchange of electronic health records of patients as part of the government's Digital India programme. 'A centralised electronic health record repository of all citizens which is the ultimate goal of the authority will ensure that the health history and status of all patients would always be available to all health institutions'. As of now, this proposal is only in the form of a concept note.

Insurance companies and health management organizations managing payments would see advantages in a singular centralized EHR, where not only the final diagnosis and outcome, but also every diagnostic and therapeutic procedure is coded for. When private purchasing agencies like insurance companies try to maximize returns, they invest considerable efforts in tracking frauds and finding technical grounds for refusing payments, also using records of patient histories with pre-existing illnesses. Under UHC, governments are encouraged to shift to the purchasing of care through insurance, while dealing with the 'moral hazards' problem characterized by liberal overconsumption of care without a sense of wrongdoing. The centralized EHR and its potential to record and make visible every health event in the population is therefore naturally attractive to government administrators, who also see value in large-scale surveillance.

However, there are various problems with this centralized EHR approach and most efforts in this direction have shown suboptimal results. One set of concerns relates to a limited ability to secure the participation and ownership of clinical users, within this 'top-down enthusiast-driven approach'. Another is the problem associated with any clean-slate approach of how to migrate historically existing records to this new system. This is not only a technical problem but an institutional one also, as there would always be a reluctance to move from working systems to something unknown. Another problem concerns the weak capacity of hospitals that are seriously overcrowded and understaffed, raising serious challenges for them to generate a list of diagnoses and aggregate statistics. Hospitals, as well as primary care providers, also vary in their level of computerization, and cannot be expected to graduate to the same level of digital capacity simultaneously. The system needs to be able to allow different providers and administrative units to make progress at their own pace. Another major issue with centralized EHR is the issue of privacy and confidentiality, and the lack of regulatory and legal frameworks in most LMICs.

Problems in shifting to a centralized EHR are not limited to LMICs and their lack of resources and capacity. One of the most recent and large-scale efforts to go down this path was by the NHS in England, losing seven billion pounds in attempting to establish a public health information architecture. Subsequently, France has abandoned similar plans (Webster 2011). In contrast, Estonia is stated to have achieved this goal and at least Australia and Austria are committed and working towards this end, while Canada and Switzerland are looking at province-level rather than national EHRs.

8.6.2 **Thinking about alternative architecture**

An alternative approach is one which is incremental and decentralized, where each administrative unit or hospital can use its preferred EHR. The central body only ensures that standards of interoperability are managed and helps providers to access records. Denmark, for example, does not have nationwide EHR, but it is mandatory for primary care practices and hospitals to use EHRs. The Danish Health Data Network acts as a data integrator to ensure interoperability. A similar situation exists in the Netherlands, where there is a national EHR, but patients need to provide explicit permission for use of their data, which is located on hospital-specific EHRs.

Incremental decentralized approaches have unique advantages in the context of LMICs. Firstly, there are multiple information systems already in place which are up and running, and there would be a strong resistance to shutting them down. In a decentralized approach they need not be shut down, but only agree to make their data available on the central system when requested. Secondly, though a centralized EHR may provide for some functions, local systems may have many features locally required that the centralized system does not provide for. Thirdly, hospitals and primary care units could adopt systems designed for their current institutional capacity, and upgrade them periodically at a convenient pace and in parallel with the growth of services. All of these systems would provide the required population-based aggregate data, but with the level of detail in patient records required by the organization. Many primary care units may prefer simple e-registers to fully fledged EHRs.

However, privacy would need to be more secure. Ownership of records would unambiguously be with the local provider, with patients having access to their information and able to authorize its sharing, even for purposes of research.

For research and public health purposes, aggregate anonymous data would need to be gained from providers. This has great implications for privacy, confidentiality, and patient autonomy, as well as the supporting regulation.

Incremental approaches are going to need enforcement of open standards, including semantic and technical frameworks to enable interoperability. This requires a strong central authority that can define and enforce these standards. In such architecture, primary care providers would compile area and population-based public health information reflecting effective coverage, and to an extent, the possible cost of care. Information from hospitals could be organized by units corresponding to primary care providers and relayed back to them for integration with the population-based database, as well as used to create disease-based registries as required. Primary care records should be available to secondary and tertiary care providers on request. Summaries of patient care provided by hospitals and consultants would need to be attached to the available primary care record, especially if the patient has come in as a referral from that level. These measures would be enough for enabling continuity of care.

The emergence of the primary care unit as the hub of compiling population-based information has the potential to facilitate inter-sectoral data convergence, if data is presented with reference to the same administrative units in all sectors—the same definitions of village, subdistrict, and district being used across sectors. CRVS information and primary healthcare information are already population based and refer to these units. It is hospital data that needs to be better aligned with the broader public health information needs. Hospitals need to be encouraged to use EHRs consistent with notified standards required for public health, and also to report information of public health importance with reference to primary care units with which they are linked. Hospitals getting reimbursement from insurance agencies or other form of partnerships with government would have a greater motivation for using EHRs, but this is currently insufficient. For public health purposes, however, aggregate figures would need to be culled out digitally from the EHRs as pertaining to the village, subdistrict, and district and matched with primary care data.

It is worth noting that in response to the scathing National Audit Office Report on the UK's National Programme for IT in the NHS, the UK Department of Health committed 'that its investments will potentially deliver value for money because reforms to the future architecture of the programme will allow many sources of information to be connected together as opposed to assuming that all relevant information will be stored in a single system' (Webster 2011, p. 1106). However, in LMICs, this remains only as a promise and potential, with lot of work required to realize this dream.

8.7 **Conclusion**

Though the needs of health information are already large, they are set to undergo an exponential increase, driven by the developing global health agenda around UHC, SDGs, and CRVS. Responding to these needs will require ways of transforming how information of public health importance is gathered from population-based surveys, primary care providers, disease surveillance systems, and hospital information systems. There would be a greater movement towards the use of EHRs which will increasingly become a key source of information for public health. However, a single centralized EHR for an entire nation may neither be feasible nor desirable. Mandating the use of EHRs universally without reference to institutional capacity and health systems contexts is unlikely to lead to effective results. There is a strong case for making the primary care provider/ unit the hub or node where information from individual case records get drawn into a population-based public health base. If every primary healthcare unit has a clearly defined set of households registered with it, and if every household is nec- essarily allocated to a primary healh care unit at least for public health purposes, then the challenge of providing the information required for measuring progress towards UHC and the SDGs is so much closer to being addressed successfully. This is a fully formalized arrangement, which makes the nature of ICT support easier to define. For a considerable period of transition, ICT systems would have to provide support even when such allocations of households to primary care providers are most incomplete—but it helps to know the direction of movement.

The CRVS as a source of public health information gains new importance and urgency with reference to these global developments. While birth regis- tration is already improving in most nations, there is a need for a a quantum leap in reliability and completion of cause-of-death reporting, and for ensuring interoperability to enable use of such information for improving public health management. Health departments and facilities need to contribute to improv- ing data collection and quality of CRVS data. All of this calls for major reforms and technical upgrade of existing CRVS systems.

A key principle being argued for by the Expanded PHI approach is to develop an architecture that is decentralized and evolving dynamically, based on mul- tiple systems and innovations happening in parallel, with strong mechanisms of governance and inter-sectoral coordination. Systems that support providers in providing better quality and continuity of care and ensure greater access and privacy to service users are also likely to yield more reliable and actionable information even at centralized levels, compared to systems that trivialize or run roughshod over these concerns.

Note

i   United Nations, General Assembly: Sixty-seventh session: Agenda item 123; Global health and foreign policy: A/67/L.36. This resolution takes care of the following: 'World Health Report 2010, entitled "Health systems financing: the path to universal coverage", and the Social Protection Floor Initiative endorsed by the United Nations Chief Executives Board for Coordination in April 2009, International and regional meetings that reaffirm the importance of universal health coverage, including the Mexico City Political Declaration on Universal Health Coverage, adopted on 2 April 2012, the Bangkok Statement on Universal Health Coverage, adopted at the Prince Mahidol Award Conference on 28 January 2012, and the Tunis Declaration on Value for Money, Sustainability and Accountability in the Health Sector, adopted on 5 July 2012'.

8.8 References

Abiiro, G., McIntyre, D. (2012). Achieving universal health care coverage: Current debates in Ghana on covering those outside the formal sector. *BMC International Health and Human Rights*, **12**:25. Available at: http://www.biomedcentral.com/1472-698X/12/25

Ahoobim, O., Altman, D., Garrett, L., Hausman, V., and Huang, Y. (2012). The New Global Health Agenda Universal Health Coverage; Council on Foreign Relations. Rockefeller Foundation.

Armstrong, T. (2012). *China's 'Floating Population'*. Available at: http://scir.org/2013/10/chinas-floating-population/

Boerma, T., Eozenou, P., Evans, D, *et al.* (2014). Monitoring progress towards universal health coverage at country and global levels. *PLoS Medicine*, **11**(9): e1001731; doi:10.1371/journal.pmed.1001731.

O'Connell, T., Rasanathan, K., Chopra, M. (2014). What does universal health coverage mean? *Lancet*, **383**(9913), 277–9.

The Economist (2015). Available at: http://www.economist.com/news/leaders/21647286-proposed-sustainable-development-goals-would-be-worse-useless-169-commandments

Gwatkin, D.R., Ergo, A. (2011). Universal health coverage: friend or foe of health equity? *Lancet* 377, 2160–1.

Nyonator, F., Ofosu, A., Segbafah, M., and d'Almeida, S. (2014). Monitoring and evaluating progress towards universal health coverage in Ghana. *PLoS Medicine*, **11**(9): e1001691.

Rodney, A., Hill, P.S. (2014). Achieving equity within universal health coverage: a narrative review of progress and resources for measuring success. *International Journal for Equity in Health*, **13**, 72. Available at: http://equityhealthj.biomedcentral.com/articles/10.1186/s12939-014-0072-8

Ng, M., Fullman, N., Dieleman, J.L., *et al.* (2014). Effective coverage: A metric for monitoring universal health coverage. *PLoS Medicine* **11**(9), e1001730. doi:10.1371/journal.pmed.1001730.

Sahay, S., Sundararaman, T., and Mukherjee, A. S. (2015). Building locally relevant models for universal health coverage and its implications for health information systems: some reflections from India. *Journal of Health Informatics in Africa*, **2**(2).

Sahay, S., and Sundararaman, T. (2015). Towards a research agenda on HIS for universal health coverage: Implications for IT4D research. International Federation of

Information Processing (IFIP) 9.4, 13th International Conference on Social Implications of Computers in Developing Countries, Colombo, Sri Lanka.

Sundararaman, T., Vaidyanathan, G., Vaishnavi., S.D, *et al.* (2014). Measuring progress towards universal health coverage:An approach in the Indian context. *Economic & Political Weekly*, **xlix** (47), 60–5.

WHO (2005). *Sustainable Health Financing, Universal Coverage, Social Health Insurance— Resolutions and Decisions Annex (WHA58/2005/REC/1), Fifty-Eighth World Health Assembly*. Geneva, Switzerland, 16–25 May 2005. Available at: http://apps.who.int/ gb/ebwha/pdf_files/WHA58-REC1/english/A58_2005_REC1-en.pdf [Last accessed 4 October 2015].

WHO (2008). *World Health Organization: World Health Report—Primary Healthcare—Now More Than Ever*. World Health Organization, Geneva, Switzerland.

WHO (2010). *World Health Report—Financing Universal Health Coverage*. World Health Organization, Geneva, Switzerland.

Webster, P.C. (2011). Centralised, nationwide electronic health records schemes under assault. *Canadian Medical Association Journal*, **183**(15), e1105–6.

WHO (2014). *Strengthening Civil Registration and Vital Statistics Systems through Innovative Approaches in the Health Sector—Guiding Principles & Good Practices*, World Health Organization, Geneva, Switzerland.

Chapter 9

Health Information Systems Governance and Standards: The Challenges of Implementation

9.1 Defining Governance

The concept of governance has posed a challenge to find a universally accepted definition both within and beyond the health domain. This is surprising, since almost all discussions on health systems informatics emphasize governance as one of its key building blocks.

The distinction between management and governance is instructive. Management is defined as the set of processes through which a given set of inputs are converted to the desired outputs—a matter of managing available resources to reach a defined set of objectives. Governance, on the other hand, defines the relationship between the owners and the organization. Governance sets the objectives and the rules of the game—at least at one level. To give an example, the governance of a corporate firm is vested with the board of directors or company board elected by its shareholders. The board then hires the chief executive, sets the goals, and defines the rules. Once this is done, the chief executive who heads the management works to efficiently mobilize and use resources, including choosing the team and devising strategies required to achieve the objectives. The board may also set certain formal and informal boundaries within which the management will act.

Despite the complexities and multidimensionality inherent to it, there is a general consensus that the governance function characterizes a set of controls and processes (customs, policies, or laws) that are formally or informally applied to distribute responsibility or accountability among actors of a given system. When one is talking of governance as related to government functions and activities, the ownership is with 'the public' or 'the people' or 'citizens'. Ownership is exercised through representative organizations and state institutions defined in a constitution. The term *governance*, as applied to public services, therefore encompasses broad systems of representation and citizen engagement, accountability, power and institutional authority, and the rule of law.

9.1.1 **Health governance and IT governance**

When discussing governance in the context of public health informatics, we have to recognize two distinct but overlapping domains: health governance and IT governance. Health governance is required to achieve health goals—defined in the World Health Report 2000 as responding to the legitimate expectations of the population, ensuring fairness of contribution, and ultimately, improving health (WHO 2000). It is the protective role of the government to ensure the best health outcomes for the population and protect its people from financial hardship, and its responsive role is to ensure that health services needed for relief from suffering and distress and preventable mortality are accessible to all.

Health governance has been defined as policy guidance to the whole health system; the coordination between actors and the regulation of different functions, levels, and actors in the system; optimally allocating resources and ensuring accountability towards all stakeholders. Although many actors have an influence on governance, there is a central role for the state in ensuring equity, efficiency, and sustainability of the health system. This requires a strong capacity at the Ministry of Health (MOH), its deconcentrated services or decentralized structures, and local governments. The health system is accountable to the population at all levels: the individual provider to the patient, and the MOH to the overall population (van Olmen *et al.* 2012).

The other governance domain is IT governance. Here the role of the government is to create the conditions for development of IT, introduce mechanisms for making choices, promote greater public access to its capabilities, ensure that there is a level playing ground for multiple providers to innovate and deliver services, protect confidentiality and privacy of individuals and organizations, and safeguard national security.

The government, acting on behalf of its citizens, fulfils obligations in these domains through its regulatory roles, its stewardship roles, and through direct provisioning of essential services. Regulation refers to the enforcement of relevant laws and rules. The term 'stewardship' has been used as almost synonymous with governance, but here we use it to refer to government actions towards steering development even by private players through policy measures and allocation of resources, which may be natural, financial, or knowledge based. Incentives, positive and negative, financial and non-financial, are major forms of exercising stewardship. But government has also what is called 'soft power'—the influence that is exercised by sheer moral persuasion linked to its legitimacy. Governments can be seen as performing their roles through 'carrots, sticks, and sermons'.

9.1.2 **Governance as power and politics**

However, the decision-making role of government is not a homogenous, uncontested technical domain based on technical merits of different options. Far from it; it is a highly contested terrain where many stakeholders with very different primary objectives, and with multiple levels of access to power and knowledge, influence decisions to tilt in their favour. One of the central functions and definitions of governance is the ability to negotiate and either win consent or enforce one option from among many.

> 'The definition of goals and the choice for a particular balance between goals reflects the interests and values of the actors that make up the health (or IT) system at the central or local level. This balance emerges from the power relations between actors and may reflect the political context and the influence of global, bilateral and other "external" actors "y"'

> (van Olmen *et al.* 2012, p. 25).

Governance is therefore the seeking of a balance, taking into account the values and principles of actors in the system through a process of negotiation based on principles of fairness. Good governance is therefore defined as a set of principles and processes that ensures this. It would include, at the least, transparency, participation, accountability, fairness, or non-discrimination, rule of law, and adherence to the larger constitutional laws and values.

9.2 **Governance in Public Health Informatics**

We can now go back over each of the challenges of public health informatics we discussed in Chapters 1–8 and map the governance role and challenges in each. Governance is a cross-cutting issue affecting all the domains discussed earlier. But there are some governance challenges, as in the development of standards or data policies, which are addressed more comprehensively in this chapter.

In Chapter 3, we discussed the constraints to the use of information. We noted that the potential for use of information for management action is highest at decentralized levels, and therefore the greater the commitment to decentralization, the greater the use of data. Centralized information systems designed with an almost exclusive focus on monitoring, as a form of vertical accountability, tend to encourage data of poor quality and discourage data use. Similarly, the less hierarchical the system and the greater its commitment to local empowerment, the higher is the likelihood of establishing conversations over data which can positively enable better data quality and use. A corollary is that information use at local levels is far more likely when stakeholders see themselves as a community of practice than as part of a command and control chain. These are all governance-related choices.

The less transparent and democratic the government, and the less given it is to the rule of law, the more it is penetrated by vested interests. This translates to greater pressures on the health information system (HIS) to become a tool for control or surveillance over populations. In response, the workforce will seek to generate only those versions of the truth as are convenient to it and to subvert the systems of control being exercised, and what they believe the 'top' wants to see.

In Chapter 4, the problematic discussed was of 'integration'. Multiple systems with different ownerships emerge rapidly, often duplicating each other, but even when under pressure to do so, they are unable to communicate with one another. Although to the lay observer the government is a homogenous monolith, in practice it is quite heterogeneous internally with multiple centres of power: different programme management divisions within each department (i.e. each disease control department, or the maternal and child health division); different departments within the government (such as for IT, health, audits, procurement, and so on); and different levels of government in a federal polity (federal, provincial, district, and local administrations). Furthermore, the government also has to negotiate a wide variety of external pressures, ranging from external donors and corporate forces, to civil society groups—each with different information requirements and priorities. Courts and the legal process can intervene in unpredictable ways. There is also a legacy that present governments inherit from the past.

Therefore, should not such multiple centres of power be fewer in less democratic or plural societies, and least in, say, military dictatorships? On the contrary, the impression we have from having worked in a large number of low and middle-income countries (LMICs) is that these problems are invariable— and perhaps more so where political power is centralized. Where processes of negotiation are explicit, transparent, and well-documented, they are likely to hold better across stakeholders, and for a longer period of time, than when decisions are pushed through by a sleight of hand, or by someone with the transient authority to ride roughshod over others' views. But negotiations in a terrain that is so technically demanding will always be characterized by high degrees of information asymmetry and uncertainties about future developments. Addressing them requires its own particular governance and institutional mechanisms.

We have discussed the problematic of integration to involve building consensus at least on three levels: creating data standards including data and metadata; creating technical standards specifying common codes of communication and storage; and, most challenging at the level of institutions, creating the readiness for them to be transparent and collaborative in their endeavours.

Other than institutional mechanisms, this multilevel integration requires a visionary leadership—ideally a democrat with necessary authority, and who exercises it judiciously. To no one's surprise, that is currently a rather tall order across most nations.

In Chapters 5 and 7, a host of new technologies related to the cloud and big data and their ensuing complexity are discussed. Here a number of new governance challenges emerge. One is reconciling potential benefits to population health, with risks to individual privacy; as technical developments continue to outpace legal advances, or even administrative and civil society's scrutiny. Many LMICs and emerging economies do not have adequate laws in place to define or safeguard privacy. Another challenge is to define ownership over data given the multiplicity of actors involved, the geographical dispersion of where the cloud is, how data is used and reused, and the ambiguity of jurisdiction. Data is often collected by an agency for one stated purpose, and then further exploited for a number of other purposes including commercial ones. The definition of ownership, and of owners' rights to data, as well as a definition of what information should mandatorily be put up on the public domain, are eminently governance functions. With respect to design of the cloud architecture and related new technologies too, government has a stewardship role– to promote technologies less susceptible to vendor lock-ins and more supportive of innovation, allow for ease of upgradation and greater degrees of participation, and above all to push for capacity development within nations so as to defend sovereignty and local ownership.

In Chapter 6, the discussion is about institutions, those of healthcare provisioning, management, policymaking, and financing. If we understand institutions as rules of the game, the pre-eminent role of governance is rule-setting and the pre-eminent rule-setter is the government. However, management of all organizations—the players of the game—need the autonomy to define their own processes and rules within a larger rule framework defined by governance. Such rules define their relationships with other organizations and boundaries within which they operate and exercise decision-making, and demarcate areas that are out of bounds. Where governments are direct service providers of health or IT services, their internal rules have a major influence on the domain, since they are by nature a large-scale monopoly on the terrain.

In Chapter 8, we have discussed the challenges of futuristic public health informatics solutions using the examples of universal health coverage (UHC) and Sustainable Development Goals (SDGs). Governance is concerned with futuristic agenda setting; defining new needs for information and technical solutions to meet those needs. Predicting the future is complex, full of risks, and definite expertise is limited. Governance then is about making technical and institutional choices where taking particular paths does not preclude other choices which may become relevant in the future.

One area of governance not discussed earlier, but which is central to the regulatory and stewardship roles of governance is the setting and implementation of IT standards, and establishing a general policy on data. Both fall more in the realm of IT governance than health governance, but with important overlaps. We discuss some of these issues in the next section.

9.3 **The Political Economy of Standards**

Standards are often perceived as some sort of pre-existing artefacts or ideals that lie in wait to be uncovered or discovered by a committee of experts. The reality is that standards are neither neutral, nor natural, nor preordained (Jolliffe 2014). They are constructed along with the rest of an organization's everyday life. Standards could perform many functions. They could facilitate interoperability, or even raise barriers of entry and limit the players. The creation of standards can only be understood like any other production—in terms of who produces what, how, why, for whom, and who gains from it. Production of standards takes place within the broader space of production of ICT and its architecture, and the systems they are part of.

To understand standards, we could consider two other usages of the word. In music, what we call a standard—a Jazz standard for example—is a set of rules, a structure within which musicians are simultaneously constrained and freed to enable collaboration and creativity. The other is the use of 'standards' as a tool in battle, where a standard is held aloft as a rallying point, with the power to make visible, sustain, and differentiate activities and interests of the group from those of the rest.

We tend to focus during discussions on the 'use value' of standards, that is, what they are used for in particular contexts. But in dominant capitalist modes of production, a standard has 'exchange value', and also 'added value' in its implementation (Jolliffe 2014). This refers to its value when it is produced as part of manufacturing a commodity for sale on the market. To give an example, Windows NT is embedded with a POSIX subsystem, since the latter is a requirement by the United States Department of Defence procurement regulations. Though with no use value, it has plenty of exchange value in the lucrative US defence market. Another example is when South Africa mandated the use of HL7 standard in its provincial hospitals. Major international vendors provided systems compliant with this standard, and in the process gained commercial advantage. But the standard was made on the grounds that it is required for hospital information systems to talk to one another—which still does not happen and has not been helped by this adoption. The governance challenge is to ensure that health IT standards provide use value in context (provide information needed for achieving health systems goals) while remaining sensitive to how they play out in the market where the policy objectives would be to ensure enough suppliers, ensure ease of procurement, and avoid unnecessary mark-up in prices.

Standards are 'de facto' or 'de jure'. De facto standards are those that have evolved due to widespread 'spontaneous' adoption, and won acceptance. These are often more important than formally approved standards. De facto standards run the risk of becoming unstable over time, and taking the status of formal standards. De jure refers to standards produced and declared by recognized agencies of governance such as 'standards development organizations', some of which are inter-government agencies such as the International Organization for Standardization (ISO), (TC 215 for clinical use, and devices later replaced by ISO/TR 14639), international organizations such as WHO and the UN (e.g. SDMX-HD), or even vendor consortiums (SNOMED and HL7). Often despite formal approval, these standards compete for market share and legitimacy with those promoted by other standards development organizations, and other de facto standards. Different institutions have roles that are intertwined and overlaid in complex ways; WHO, HL7, and IHE each have 'category A' liaison status within ISO. ISO sets many of the rules of this game, and it requires experience, skills, and influence (and sometimes brute force) to effectively manipulate the standards that emerge from their interaction.

Within health IT, a big debate concerns open vs. proprietary standards. Open standards are linked to—but not to be confused with—open source, and relate to access and transparency provided for with due process. Standards attracting intellectual property rights are excluded from this definition, but many standards organizations do not insist on this understanding. Today formal standards are vying for a position to support the development of architecture of information systems such as related to health insurance exchange (HIX), electronic medical records (EMR), health information exchange (HIE), and health insurance exchange (HIX) identifiers, and various others related to mobile data and cloud-based services. Each needs a cluster of standards to promote its development and use.

One interesting case study was the attempt by WHO to produce a standard (called the SDMX-HD) for the exchange of aggregate health data and its indicators. While being of significant interest to public health informatics, the process of evolving this standard has stalled over the last few years, and is now being replaced by a new standard called ADX (Aggregate Data Exchange), which is being developed by the Quality Research and Public Health (QRPH) technical committee within the 'Integrating the Health Enterprise' (IHE) consortium. The rationale for embarking on this effort was driven by a number of factors.

Despite the enormous interest in, and appetite for, EMR patient-based systems, such systems are still not widespread across many countries—particularly the resource constrained countries across Africa and Asia. So the dominant form of health information collection and exchange is aggregate data (How many births? How many deaths? How many malaria cases?). These aggregate data elements are collected and further aggregated across time and space, and typically divided by denominators to create health indicators. The generation, processing, presenting, and responding to such indicators provides the engine of health systems management on the different administrative levels of many countries. Whereas the e-health standards processes of Organisation for Economic Co-operation and Development (OECD) countries have reflected the dominant reality in those countries—an ever-increasing uptake of EMR systems generating patient data, which then needs to be exchanged for various purposes—the widespread flow of aggregate data, which has typically not originated in an EMR, has largely been ignored by the major e-health standards consortiums. Standards are typically developed by committees of experts, representing vendors with a direct interest in the outcome of the process; or they are built by consultants whose intimate knowledge of the standards places them in an advantageous position in the market. And so the standards which are developed tend to reflect the guiding market forces—where is the money to be made (OECD countries); and what are the standards which have the greatest market exchange value (those which interface with EMR systems).

A flurry of recent activity at WHO[1] over the past three years has increased the pressure on all countries to adopt e-health standards and develop HIE architectures. Yet neither WHO nor any of the standards consortiums and standards development organizations have produced standards which focus on the dominant health information exchange in the global south. SDMX-HD was an attempt to address the gap, but its demise reflected a fundamental reorientation of WHO's role regarding standards. Without the experience, expertise, structures, or political will to *develop* e-health standards, they took on a new posture of advocating market-based best practices as (supposedly) embodied in international standards.

ADX was conceived in response to this direction as an effort to standardize the existing concrete reality of aggregate health data exchange in the global south within a formal process and maintenance body. That is, to place such data exchange on a formal footing by working through a globally recognized maintenance agency (IHE) with a formal balloting, testing, and publication process in collaboration with CDC (Centers for Disease Control and Prevention, USA) and other FOSS (Free and Open Source Software) groupings clustered under the openHIE umbrella.

Strictly speaking, IHE does not create standards, but rather profiles existing standards. So ADX is more properly described as an IHE profile than a standard as such, though from the perspective of developers, integrators, and those involved in health IT governance, the difference is not significant. ADX is currently published for trial implementation, and was tested for compliance at an integration event organized by IHE called the North American Connectathon in January 2016.

At the time of writing this book, it is still too early to say how successful or otherwise ADX will be. There are certainly some causes for concern. Despite the genuine openness of IHE as an organization towards taking on this work it is quite different to the bulk of their existing work—which profiles HL7 standards for use in the US and EU markets. The bi-annual face to face meetings are all held in the US and Europe—reflecting naturally the majority of participants. The connectathons are currently held in the United States and Europe making them quite expensive for vendors from the south to participate fully, if at all. There is also some unease within the technical committee of the market value of the ADX work. As a private sector consortium, their production activity is naturally driven by maximizing exchange value for their members. ADX, though it may have tremendous use value, is unlikely to be a money spinner.

But there are also a number of good reasons for optimism. The work is grounded in good empirical knowledge and experience of the domain. It has enthusiastic support from a number of major players in the global health arena, including HISP, CDC, and PEPFAR. It is new ground for many. For FOSS developers—for example of the DHIS 2 project—it is challenging, but also enriching to participate in the formal processes of a standards committee. For IHE there is an opportunity to extend their reputation into many countries outside of their core markets.

But the pressures do not end with a single effort—they never do. The communities of practice around open source actively engage with standards setting institutions. But analogous to the 'market' failure in public health, public health standards will not evolve as readily as open standards in other areas. A similar movement in public health informatics is required to lobby and actively engage with policy makers and standards producers and promoters to ensure that context-sensitive use value is being created, which public health informatics can use.

In Case Studies 9.1 and 9.2 we discuss national-level efforts to establish health data standards by two Asian countries.

Case Study 9.1 Setting IT Health Data Standards Setting in India

The National Rural Health Mission (NRHM) catalysed the use of HIS in the public health system. The period from 2005 to 2012 marked the design, implementation, and use of various information systems for health management information systems (HMIS), disease surveillance, mother and child tracking, immunization, human resources, e-tendering and procurements, drugs and logistics, and many more. As a result, the need for integration and standardization was deemed necessary for integrated information use and this was articulated in the 12th Plan.

The immediate post-plan period saw two standards committees in operation. First was a committee for standards for electronic health records, which was already operational since 2010, but which was expedited by the setting up of another committee in 2013. The other committee was the MDDS (Metadata and Data Standards) set up in 2013 by the Ministry of Communication and Technologies under the National e-Governance Plan (NeGP). The intent was to promote e-Governance within the country by establishing interoperability across various applications. Under MDDS, various domain-specific committees were constituted in priority areas. The Health Domain MDDS Committee was one such initiative, constituted in September 2012, under the chairmanship of a ministry joint secretary to help solve the problem of using multiple systems for the same purpose. One immediate stimulus to setting it up was that there were two systems operational for maternal and child health within the ministry: the Mother and Child Tracking System and the earlier HMIS. These two systems contained large amounts of overlapping data, but were unable to communicate with one another and provided two completely different numbers at every level.

The exercise yielded approximately 140 code directories and 1000 data elements, which were regrouped and formatted into 39 entities. These data elements would serve as the common minimum data elements for the development of IT applications for various health subdomains to facilitate interoperability among various applications. The MDDS did considerable innovative and pioneering work in listing common data elements, keeping the patient–provider relationship as central and using an appropriate ISO standard (ISO/IEC 11179) to define conceptual and value domains for each. The MDDS draft standard was made available on the ministry website for comments, but nearly two years after its submission, still remains in the draft status. This delay was due to opposition to such standards from industry elements who had a relatively good position in the government market. Furthermore, administrators lacked the confidence to take a decision where technical experts had conflicting views. Even if there were clear and obvious conflict of interest, industry spokespersons had a higher prestige and intellectual hegemony than the academics.

Stimulated by the initiation of the MDDS committee, the EHR committee finalized its recommendations in September 2014, relating primarily to the private sector, which had a larger voice in that committee. The committee ignored aggregate data, and its recommendations included a list of standards that was so wide that it made little difference to practice. It however raised a sharp debate over the decision to adopt the SNOMED CT system. Despite considerable internal opposition, the decision to adopt it prevailed and the government paid a licence fee of INR 60 million to acquire it. Potentially, universal use of SNOMED CT can make for easier integration of Indian health insurance and hospital data into the global healthcare industry, especially in the United States, but it is hardly a priority for the development of public health informatics in India. To enforce implementation, the central government sent letters to the states asking them to ensure all software complied with SNOMED CT standards, without providing clarity on what this meant or the costs involved. Perception of what implementing EHR standards means has become centred around adoption of SNOMED CT—but that is not likely to happen anytime soon. Meanwhile the objective of interoperability, at least between the two systems dedicated largely to maternal and child health within the same department, remains as distant as ever and work on integration across multiple systems continues to remain a dream.

9.3.1 Governance of IT standards

The problem illustrated in Case Study 9.1 is not unique; indeed, it is almost universal. It draws attention to the fact that creating standards is not an end in itself, but requires mechanisms to ensure that they serve the purpose for which they are intended. Furthermore, while publication of standards is necessary, it is not sufficient, since the ways to implement them are not obvious. There is a whole institutional framework that needs to be created, with multiple possibilities of failure. In addition, it is exchange value and not use value that drives what is prioritized in the development of standards. Standards with high monetary value and industry possibilities get an emphasis even if few can use them, while much more immediate, urgent, and feasible concerns of public health get relegated to the back seat.

Adjudication between technical contentions, especially where multibillion dollar corporate stakes are in contention, is not easy. This requires separate institutions for governance, which set responsibility for oversight to act, remove, or reward as based on performance. That body should be independent from management and represent the principles the organization serves—the public interest in better health outcomes. In not-for-profit organizations, governance is usually based on the identification of individuals who by their work and actions are judged capable of furthering the goals of that organization. But IT in healthcare is a huge profit and growth industry—there are issues which cannot be settled by identification of few leaders at the top, and it is not possible to find a person suitable on all counts.

An effective body for setting standards or for overseeing their implementation has to contend with politics based both upon the desire to act for the public good, and negotiating through the different political and commercial interests. There is a huge potential for conflict of interest when certain actions are required that may not be interpreted with public acclaim, or may face opposition from other powerful interest groups. This is where the provision of health services in many LMICs runs into problems, because the governance structure is often flawed, allowing for a poor awareness of the conflicts of interests, and insufficient capacity and autonomy to negotiate the political requirements with the larger public interests in mind.

IT governance is defined 'as the processes that ensure the effective and efficient use of IT in enabling an organization to achieve its goals'[2]. Here the organization could be a commercial corporate body, a non-profit autonomous institution set up and acting on behalf of the government or industry, or a government department. Given the complexity of requirements of IT governance, especially the very rapid changes that developments in technology bring about, and also given the familiarity of the IT sector with standards development, it is not surprising that standards for IT governance is a significant area of their emphasis.

9.4 **Standards for IT Governance**

One of the first efforts in this regard was in the United Kingdom, where the ISO 38500 was established in 2008 as the British standard for 'Corporate Governance of Information Technology' (ISO 2008). The framework comprised definitions, principles, and a model. The standard set out six principles for good corporate governance of IT:

i)   Responsibility
ii) Strategy

iii) Acquisition
iv) Performance
v) Conformance
vi) Human behaviour

It also provided guidance to those advising, informing, or assisting directors of health IT systems. Another important development in ISO-based standards was ISO/TR 14639-1:2012 (ISO 2012) which aimed to identify the business requirements of e-health architecture, as well as provide a generic and comprehensive context description to inform architectural structuring of HIS. Another set of standards for IT governance is the COBIT 5, a framework developed for the governance and management of enterprise IT (ISACA 2012).

We next present Case Study 9.2 from the Philippines where an e-governance approach based on COBIT was adopted.

9.4.1 Learnings from the Philippines case study

The Philippines case emphasizes that developing a national e-health strategy is founded on strong governance and leadership. Orchestration of the many stakeholders with competing agendas through an accepted leadership framework and an accessible health information exchange is key to this integration. The adoption of suitable IT governance standards allows a government to map out all the necessary institutional structures and organizational capacities for IT governance—both existing and desirable, and then move systematically towards closing the gaps. Another learning is the importance given to articulating the health sector performance improvements that the introduction of IT is expected to facilitate. Yet another lesson is that given the complexities and the multiplicity of stakeholders, different institutions are needed for negotiating with and bringing all on board. Thus institutions emerge for writing and renewing standards and others for implementation—and yet others for monitoring.

9.5 Creating New Institutions

Governments hesitate to create new institutions, often due to the poor performance of existing ones. Also there is the active resistance of existing institutions to the rise of new ones. The expenditure on infrastructure and administration implied in the creation of a new institution is also a reason for this hesitation. But IT governance and IT in healthcare is a new area, and to some extent, new institutions are inevitable. The way forward is to learn from the past experiences of both well-performing and poorly performing governance institutions to design the new.

(continued on page 228)

Case Study 9.2 Governance and Architecture for National e-Health Programmes: The Philippines

Origins

The Department of Health of the Republic of the Philippines released a national e-health strategy in October 2010, which identified five key result areas encompassing a wide range of national HIS. Initially, not many were aware of it, nor were involved in its development. Hence it remained largely a policy intention. In July 2012, the WHO and the International Telecommunications Union launched the WHO-ITU National e-Health Strategy Development Programme that aimed to share 'experiences and lessons learned from national e-health strategy development efforts and identify stakeholders (donors, international/regional organizations, Ministries of Health/ICT) roles in supporting national e-health strategy development'. At the first Asia e-Health Information Network general meeting in Bangkok in August 2012, twenty countries participated in the regional dissemination of a toolkit developed by this programme.

Guided by the toolkit, the Philippines Department of Health (DOH) together with the Department of Science and Technology (DOST) released a Joint Memorandum creating the National e-Health Governance Steering Committee and Technical Working Group. This body established the decision-making framework for e-health matters of national scale. The Steering Committee was composed of the secretaries of the DOH and DOST, and it included the president and CEO of the Philippine Health Insurance Corporation, the Commission on Higher Education, the University of the Philippines, Manila, and the National University of Health Sciences. With this mandate, and the tool kit, the Technical Working Group revised the 2010 national e-health strategy and the resulting document as 'The Philippine eHealth Strategic Framework and Plan 2013–2020 (PeHSFP)'.

Triggers and Pain Points

The PeHSFP came at a time when the demand for better information was increasing from various stakeholders. While global agencies asked for information to measure progress towards the Millennium Development Goals, new developments in technology exerted pressure on government and private corporations such as mobile health, privacy, and telemedicine.

In addition, the Department of Budget and Management, in an effort to optimize government's IT investments, released the Medium-term IT Harmonization Initiative (MITHI), which encouraged government agencies to collaborate and consolidate resources around a shared infrastructure (iGov) and make seamless services available to the citizens. All these developments were coming in rapid succession, making it difficult for the heads of agencies—who had minimal or no technical background—to understand how they could provide direction to their respective management teams.

Adopting an IT Governance Framework

At the first meeting of the National e-Health Steering Committee, the members approved the Philippine 'eHealth Strategic Framework and Plan'. Faced with multimillion investments from MITHI (trigger point) and the complexity of the fragmented and multistakeholder environment of the health sector (pain point), they resolved to adopt an IT governance framework to organize and systematize how investments should be made to ensure that health benefits are realized by the people. To enable this, the Steering Committee decided to adopt COBIT 5—a business framework for the governance and management of enterprise IT. With this decision, the Steering Committee took accountability for the national e-health programme and provided four strategic directions to the Technical Working Group:

i) Decrease maternal deaths to less than 50 per 100,000 live births
ii) Increase universal health coverage to over 50 per cent of Filipinos
iii) Complete the health facility enhancement programme
iv) Use information technology in all government health facilities

Given these priorities, the TWG aligned, planned, and organized their activities to ensure the delivery of the benefits to the citizenry. In their preliminary discussions, they agreed that the most cost-effective approach to integrating the fragmented health system was to establish the Philippine Health Information Exchange (PHIE) to serve as the connector to all stakeholders of the health system. The PHIE was conceptualized as an open architecture that contained core registries and standards to inform public and private information systems on how to interact securely and effectively with each other. With investments from WHO, a series of consultations were made to build capacity for the TWG to build, acquire, and implement the PHIE.

Expert Groups

The WHO-ITU National e-Health Strategy Toolkit listed the following seven core components of a comprehensive programme:

i)   Leadership and governance
ii) Strategy and investment
iii) Services and applications
iv) Standards and interoperability
v)   Infrastructure
vi) Legislation, policy, and compliance, and
vii) Workforce

'Leadership and governance' was emphasized as the most important component and one that encompassed and enabled the rest. In their initial meetings, the TWG realized that they did not have expertise on 'Standards and interoperability'. Upon review of the component 'Legislation, policy, and compliance', the TWG identified the Data Privacy Act of 2012 as a significant regulation that will have an impact on health information management in the country. Cognizant of the toolkit framework and the current deficiency in capabilities on its certain aspects, the TWG approved the creation of the Health Data Standards Expert Group and the Health Data Privacy Expert Group. This was consistent with the recommendation of the Toolkit: 'The governance structure and roles should be set up early in the vision development process to gain credibility, coordinate efforts and establish the necessary expert and reference groups'.

Once convened, the Health Data Standards Expert Group immediately started work on stakeholder mapping and identified entities crucial to the standards development process. This resulted in a Standards Change Management Manual that defined how standards are proposed, deliberated, approved or rejected, and formally entered in a standards catalogue. The Health Data Privacy Expert Group, on the other hand, began working on a framework for complying with the Data Privacy Act of 2012, but also encouraging sharing of health data. This involved extensive consultation with the relevant stakeholders and the formulation of privacy guidelines for health data and a consent framework.

Other Expert Groups

As the engagement of the TWG progressed, issues were raised and agreements were reached to create expert groups to address them. Some of these expert groups were: the Advisers Group (private sector); the Health Enterprise Architecture Expert Group; the Risk Management Expert Group; the Finance and Sustainability Expert Group; the Capacity Building task force; and the EMR group.

Data Sharing Agreements

Constrained with the draft privacy guidelines, the Department of Health, the Philippine Health Insurance Corporation, and the Department of Science and Technology worked on a data sharing agreement to describe how the agencies will collaborate around the PHIE.

Monitoring and Evaluation

More recently, the TWG created the Monitoring and Evaluation Expert Group to measure the performance of the Philippine e-Health Strategic Framework and Plan.

Figure 9.1 shows the schematic summarizing the structures established by the TWG.

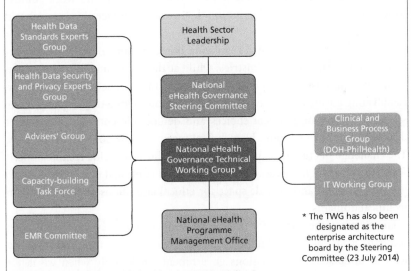

Fig. 9.1 Structures established by the TWG, Philippines.

If we look at the Philippines case study, we see three types of institutions. First are those having authority—whose decisions are, by definition, the decisions of the government in this arena. These are the regulatory and policy-making institutions, such as the National e-Health Steering Committee and the Technical Working Group. Second are institutions which are essentially for deciding on technical matters and providing space for considerable negotiation at the technical levels. These are expert committees, task forces, and working groups. And third are executive organizations like the programme management groups—those which undertake contracting and financing for implementation, and others which undertake inspections and certification for licensing and compliance with standards.

Each institution needs to derive its mandate and its governing body from legal authority: laws that are passed by parliament or rules approved by cabinet and ministry. These rules inform organizations of their turf, and what powers they have. Once this is in place, the governing board passes its powers on to management, or an executive who in turn provides the rules and organization of work processes, and implements the human resources and knowledge management policies that are most suited for effective and efficient services. Get these right, couple it with good leadership and work culture, would potentially create an institution that works. However, this is easier said than done.

The challenge in establishing regulatory bodies is how to build in accountability to parliament and ministries, while at the same time providing them with the required autonomy and freedom from interference. The challenge in establishing governing bodies for policy is acknowledging the need to provide space for legitimate political choices and democratic consultations, yet let decisions be informed more by technical merit than by political expediency. The challenge in creating expert committees is how to decide technical merit when there are high degrees of uncertainty and contested evidence, and also how to recognize and provide space for ethical and philosophical choices in technical domains.

For example, the choice for or against an open source system, or an open standard, is as much a value-based political choice, as a technical one, and we can understand the decisions governments make only when we factor in both. Another example is of the United States where, to promote compliance to standards, the government has undertaken to underwrite the costs of adoption of new standards with substantial financial incentives (Centres for Medicare and Medicaid Services 2015). Most LMICs would find it neither feasible nor desirable to do so. However, in LMICs like the Philippines, if the public providers all move into the new standards, the private sector would find it advantageous to follow suit. The approach chosen is again a political choice, which is often fraught with long delays.

Are there ways to remove influence of vested interests and short-term political expediency from decision-making in governance? Removing obvious conflict of interests in the decision-making process usually correlates with more independent decisions. Allowing for a separation between the technical advisory institution and the decision-making and implementation bodies is another. A good example of an institution designed to negotiate the complex minefield of the technical, political, and ethical is the National Institute of Clinical Excellence (NICE) in the United Kingdom. Its mandate is to recommend various procedures and therapies that can be included as part of the UK's National Health Service (NHS), and to prescribe and disseminate the standard treatment guidelines and their quality guidelines. Whenever new therapies become available for inclusion, NHS refers the question to NICE, which subsequently calls for expert volunteers and a chairperson. From those who volunteer, a screening committee selects the most suitable representative. Civil society groups and patient groups also get representation. All committee members and experts are provided training on the complexities of technical decision-making and the process that NICE has instituted. A background note of minimum evidence standards, data use, cost-effectiveness, and safety is presented to the committee along with member comments. The response or reply to every criticism made has to be articulated and recorded and after taking it all into account, the document is revised. Often voting is held to arrive at the final decision.

It is worth noting that the process is so robust that many pharmaceuticals of doubtful reliability would rather not present their case than have it busted here. NICE has now acquired such credibility that both professionals and public respect it equally. And despite a fair number of legal contestations, there is not a single instance of a court having overturned a NICE decision.

Any institution of IT governance will have to contend with not only the issue of defining standards, but also of data policy. This includes areas like data ownership, data storage, data retrieval, and use of information. It will also have to decide on how to certify compliance with standards and incentives for compliance, and the penalties or dis-incentives for non-compliance. It will have to protect against monopoly control and vendor lock-ins, and also recommend policies related to procurement of service providers and IT developers. It will need to have methods and tools for evaluation of products in the context of its use. Though standards like COBIT 5 map this entire area and provide standards, the institutional mechanisms by which these standards can be agreed upon and implemented require an understanding of the political economy of not only the standards—but also of institutions of governance.

9.6 **Bottom-up Governance**

The Philippines is an example of best practice in the area of public health informatics governance, but clearly many LMICs have many miles to go before they reach there. Where practitioners have little influence on decision-making and where a few monopoly players have all the political influence, it could be frustrating to try for change at the top—however essential this may be. Often administrators are convinced at a personal level, but it is asking a lot of an individual administrator to set up such elaborate institutions as the Philippines E- Health Authority and NICE. We argue for a combination of both. There are no rewards for administrators to take the risks of pushing such reform, and politicians combining in themselves an inability to grasp technical detail with a susceptibility to vested interests would not push for it either. How one can move forward in such circumstances is a question many LMICs have not yet found an answer to.

There has to be a way of engaging with the issue to enable more and more persons to appreciate the political choices that need to be made, and also to evolve the technical solutions required. The experts need to create networks among themselves so that when the political window of opportunity opens, one can make the best use of it. One way to strengthen communities of practice across different programmes and providers is to show how there could be bottom standards to help solve some of these apparently wicked integration problems of public health informatics.

In Case Study 9.3 we discuss the bottom-up standards development attempted in Bihar, India.

9.7 **Conclusion**

A key recommendation with respect to HIS always concerns the governance of data, project management, and design and implementation of standards. As the future becomes increasingly uncertain and unclear, governance becomes a key issue as this function is responsible for making strategic choices and putting in place an implementation framework.

Most LMICs are currently grappling with governance issues and governance design. One way forward is to develop and use governance standards as a way of negotiating the complexity of governance requirements. This is more than just establishing ad hoc technical committees and developing blueprints to implement different options—it is designing an entire governance architecture. The most successful example among LMICs is of the Philippines, but there are fairly good examples in developed nations like Canada and Australia as well.

Case Study 9.3 Solving an Interoperability Problem at the Local Level—between HR HIS and HMIS in Bihar, India

One interesting example of bottom-up local standards development is the efforts to integrate interoperability between a human resources management information system (called iHRIS) and the HMIS in one province of India. The technical collaborators were IntraHealth International, in collaboration with the National Health Systems Resource Centre (NHSRC) and HISP India. The governance institution was the State Health Society, Bihar (SHSB). Being a very local development, this did not attract any of the attention and contestations that large-scale national-level integration efforts attract. It was also positioned as a problem-solving exercise, not as a governance reform instrument. The purpose of integration was defined as providing for comparison and analysis of human resource data with service delivery data for decision-making. It was hoped that through this initiative, programme planning and management especially with respect to human resource allocation would improve and the information could be used for providing incentives to the workforce.

The work involved mapping common data elements and standardizing their definitions, organization unit hierarchies, exchanging data using specific solutions, and comparing and analysing cross-cutting information using combined dashboards to support decision-making. Integration involved integrating the DHIS 2 with iHRIS for manpower planning and improved service delivery—but more important was to build an alliance of like-minded practitioners and policy makers who now understood what policy changes were needed and the advantages of such architecture. There were also issues of hosting the interoperable application, allowing user level authentication for both system users (who? for what? how much?) and then negotiating a solution. This is work in progress—and very much a local experiment—but there is progress. But that is much more than can be said about efforts at the federal level.

To date, various challenges have been experienced in this modest effort at interoperability. Different departments maintain the HR HMIS and HMIS, namely the Department of Health for the HR HMIS and the State Health Society for HMIS. Due to this different ownership of systems, large mismatches were found in the organization unit hierarchies in terms of nomenclature, facility type, and upgradation status, and the geographical location within the state. It became a huge challenge to synchronize and create a standard hierarchy of the service delivery points in both the systems, and visualize how such changes would be synched in the future.

The HR HMIS and the HMIS had fundamental differences in their system design. On the one hand, the HR HMIS has the focus on the human resource information, deployments, and payroll management, which includes data on human resources deployed at all service delivery as well as the administrative offices. In contrast, the HMIS has the data only for the service delivery points in the structure. Therefore, it required creation of different groups within the DHIS 2, which could differentiate employees, deployed at service delivery organizations within a district, and those deployed at administrative offices.

Eventually one could make the two systems talk to each other. But the challenges remain. The implementation of such an interoperable application requires a greater ownership of both parties in terms of maintenance of the system once it is put in use—and it is difficult to ensure it with a policy support. Another key area of collaboration is to maintain a master facility list which can take changes from both systems and maintains data integrity. This central mechanism has been difficult to create for institutional reasons. Yet what this example shows is that while one is waiting for the big changes to happen, there are many things that can be done and learned from by building interoperabilities around specific needs and uses at the local level. Even at the national level, two programme managers deciding to work together can make their systems more interoperable if they better understand the barriers.

One could begin at the top like the Philippines did, but one has to be cautioned that many other nations that began at the top have not necessarily succeeded, or at least, not as yet—as the Indian case study shows. Efforts for reform at the top have to be complemented by communities of practice that work on bottom-up reforms. Bottom-up approaches to managing HIS data and strengthening local mechanisms to enable compliance to standards are useful for improving everyday work in implementation and to build understanding among partners.

It is not our contention that without a policy decision at the top, field-level initiatives can scale up or even sustain. However, communities of practice get sensitized to the big issues through their active engagement with the problems and this understanding diffuses into policymaking circles and exists at its margins. At times when there is a crisis—perhaps a parliamentary committee inquiring into non-performance, a media story, or an opportunity like a new leadership wanting to make a difference—this understanding that has been incubated in a local context could get mainstreamed.

The need is therefore to build an understanding of governance that takes an inclusive 'public health informatics' perspective, rather than one which is primarily technical. Whereas industry is almost always conscious of how technical choices will impact its profits, other stakeholders—especially those working for equity in healthcare—are much less sensitive to the way apparently value-neutral technical choices could adversely impact the goals that they work for. Governance is required to make political choices with respect to standards and the design of agencies (institutions) setting up and implementing those standards. These choices must emphasize the 'use values' related to public health goals, rather than the 'exchange values' related to industry profits. The governance capacity to make 'politically correct technical choices' requires an enabling policy environment, which is consultative and supportive, constructive and creative, and does not intervene in everyday work. Governance capacity requires clarity about the multiple expectations from IT that different stakeholders in the health sector have, and mechanisms by which conflicting interests can be negotiated without compromising core values of public health related to equity and participation, and without any loss of effectiveness or efficiency.

Given the well-known contemporary problems of governance in LMICs, this is asking a lot of governance. But there is reason for hope. Most governments are seized by these problems, and as communities of practice widen their presence and influence, more positive case studies are sure to emerge—until a trend is established.

Acknowledgements

Section 9.3 on the political economy of standards has borrowed considerably from the notes taken of a lecture delivered by Dr Bob Jolliffe at a seminar in Center for Technology and Policy, IIT, Chennai held in 2014. We gratefully acknowledge the contribution.

Case Study 9.2 is based on a note by Alvin B. Marcelo, MD, Associate Professor of Surgery and Health Informatics, University of the Philippines Manila, and member of the national e-health governance Technical Working Group (TWG) and adviser to the national e-health governance Steering Committee. We gratefully acknowledge the contribution.

Notes

1. For example, the January 2014 Forum on e-Health Standardization and Interoperability (http://www.who.int/ehealth/events/final_forum_report.pdf)

2. Gartner IT glossary—http://www.gartner.com/it-glossary/it-governance

9.8 **References**

Centres for Medicare and Medicaid services (2015). Electronic Health Records (EHR) Incentive Programs [Online]. Available at: https://www.cms.gov/Regulations-and-Guidance/Legislation/EHRIncentivePrograms/index.html?redirect=/ehrincentiveprograms [Accessed 6 October 2015].

International Organization for Standardization (ISO) (2008). International Standard ISO/IEC 38500: Corporate governance of information technology. [Online]. Available at: http:/www.iso.org/ [Accessed 6 October 2015].

International Organization for Standardization (ISO) (2012). ISO/TR 14639-1:2012—Health informatics—Capacity-based eHealth architecture roadmap—Part 1: Overview of national eHealth initiatives [Online]. Available at: http://www.iso.org/iso/catalogue_detail?csnumber=54902 [Accessed 6 October 2015].

ISACA (2012). COBIT 5: A Business Framework for the Governance and Management of Enterprise IT [Online]. Available at: http://www.isaca.org/COBIT/Pages/default.aspx [Accessed 6 October 2015].

Jolliffe, B. (2014). The Production of Global Health IT Standards, Presentation for the meeting on 'International seminar on building communities of practice to strengthen capacities around public health information systems', Chennai, India, 1–3 October 2014.

van Olmen, J., Criel, B., Van Damme, W., *et al.* (2012); *Analysing Health Systems Dynamics. A framework* (2nd edition). Studies in Health Services Organisation & Policy, 28, Antwerp, Belgium.

World Health Organization (2000). The World Health Report 2000: health systems: improving performance. World Health Organization, Geneva, Switzerland.

Chapter 10

Strengthening Healthcare Systems and Health Information Systems: Building Synergies

10.1 Introduction

In this concluding chapter, we try to place national health information systems (HIS) strengthening efforts in the context of ongoing processes of health reforms and emerging health policies at global, regional, and country levels. The aim is to understand how stronger synergies can be developed between these two sets of processes, which historically have remained relatively independent and lost opportunities for both. HIS strengthening requires an injection of appropriate policy resources, and also HIS needs to contribute to the effective materialization of the reforms themselves.

This chapter is divided into three sections. In the first, we discuss some of the contemporary health reforms initiatives that regions and countries are engaged with, and their implications for HIS. In the following section, we discuss normatively the synergies that need to be developed between the two. And finally, we conclude with an understanding of the way forward to make HIS more effective so that it can help transform health sector performance. The way forward is not only in terms of policy and implementation, but also in academia and the networking of communities engaged with health systems and HIS change.

10.2 Health Reforms and Potential Implications on National Health Information Systems

The global, regional, and national health context is rapidly changing, bringing with it many new challenges, and also expanding and revising existing ones. Whereas in the 1990s health sector reform was largely about choosing a very selective package of services based on technical measures of cost-effectiveness delivered through vertical strategies, today the emphasis is on horizontal integration, with more comprehensively defined essential health packages. With the rise of universal health coverage (UHC) as the defining discourse, the elimination of all catastrophic health expenditure becomes a priority, in addition to enabling universal access to quality healthcare. This requires matching strategies with respect to human resources for health, access to healthcare technologies, and engagement with the private health sector, all key components of contemporary health sector reform.

The World Health Organization (WHO) has repeatedly emphasized that there is no one way to achieve UHC and nations need to work out their own road maps and strategies for health systems strengthening, including optimal utilization of resources. Whatever the road map chosen, strengthening of the public health informatics (PHI) component remains at the core.

Most low and middle-income countries (LMICs) are currently engaged with strengthening their national HIS, closing the gaps in current data flows, and improving the quality and timeliness of reporting based on modern technical solutions. As discussed in this book, these efforts are seized with the problems of lack of integration of data flows, fragmentation, and also duplications in data collection. Furthermore, there are major gaps observed in cause-specific mortality and health facility records, in conducting health surveys, and getting quality data at appropriate levels of disaggregation (by age, gender, location, and socio-economic status). There are important variations in country estimates with those of regional and global organizations, raising the need for strong coordination mechanisms enabled by policy. As noted by the Regional Director, WHO, EMRO: 'In discussions with Member States, coordination and strengthening collaboration in the development and reporting of estimates emerged as key priorities and will receive focus in 2013' (WHO 2012, EMRO, Annual Report, p. 12).

There is thus need for building a seamless continuity between efforts towards improving HIS and health reforms. Development of effective HIS to support UHC is not just a matter of appropriate HIS design, but requires institutional restructuring that must come through policy efforts mandated by health reform agendas. Similarly, incorporating data on non-communicable diseases, currently ignored by routine HIS in most LMICs, requires similar policy efforts, which would then reduce the dependence on expensive and infrequent surveys. Governance reforms must address specific issues relating to IT infrastructure such as cloud hosting policies, data regulation, last mile connectivity, and various others. If such issues are directly made the subject of reform, they could more effectively strengthen national HIS, which in turn can help improve the efficacy of the reforms themselves.

In Chapter 8, we discussed at length two developments in global health which have implications for HIS strengthening—the commitment to UHC and the post-2015 SDGs. We flag in the following section a larger and more comprehensive list of such recent 'agenda-setting in global health' that places demand on public HIS.

10.2.1 The path to universal health coverage

The United Nations unanimously adopted a resolution on 12 December 2012, urging 'governments to move towards providing all people with access to affordable, quality healthcare services. It recognizes the role of health in achieving international development goals and calls for countries, civil society and international organizations to include *universal health coverage (UHC)* in the international development agenda' (United Nations 2012, p. 5).

UHC is an important global, regional, and national priority, and is linked with strategies for health financing structures and health systems strengthening. Most countries have now passed resolutions endorsing roadmaps towards boosting UHC, which will necessarily require revamping existing HIS, including the capabilities of recording financial information and tracking individual encounter-based health information disaggregated at a suitable level to monitor equity. A number of key indicators required for UHC will need to come from non-HMIS sources; raising the need for stronger technical and institutional coordination across sectors.

10.2.2 Improvement of civil registration and vital statistics systems

This initiative is also linked to the global United Nations' Commission on Information and Accountability (CoIA) for Women's and Children's Health. Its first recommendation is on vital events. To quote: 'By 2015, all countries have taken significant steps to establish a system for registration of births, deaths and causes of death, and have well-functioning health information systems that combine data from facilities, administrative sources and surveys' (Commission on Information and Accountability for Women's and Children's Health 2012). While historically, HIS in LMICs have been aggregate/statistics-based, building and strengthening civil registration and vital statistics systems (CRVS) systems will require a greater focus on individual names and vital events, and building synergies between HIS and CRVS.

10.2.3 Accelerating the Expanded Programme on Immunization to meet global and regional targets

Under the Expanded Programme on Immunization (EPI) specific priorities exist, such as the introduction of new vaccines, expanding coverage of DPT-2, and the elimination of measles. The introduction of new vaccines will require the integration of information from a cold chain with service coverage to better compare capacities for the storage and service delivery of vaccine usage. This requires the HIS to provide data at detailed levels of granularity to enable monitoring of vaccine coverage, points of dropouts, and more location-specific information on where these dropouts are taking place.

10.2.4 Saving the lives of mothers and children

Globally, there is recognition of urgent and collective efforts between countries and partners to reduce deaths among mothers and children, especially in the high burden countries. The 'Maternal Death Surveillance and Response—technical guidance' emphasizes the need for systematic and continuous surveillance of maternal deaths by linking the HIS, as well as standardized response systems and quality improvement processes from local to national levels, including the implementation and monitoring of recommendations which arise from death reviews (The Partnership for Maternal, Newborn and Child Health 2013). This is inter-related to the challenges of strengthening vital statistics, improving quality of data, improving logistic information systems to support availability of life-saving commodities, and making available data at disaggregated levels of the individual and their encounters with the health system.

10.2.5 Monitoring the core set of indicators

At the international level, preparatory to the process of evolving the post-2015 goals, the global health institutions arrived at a consensus 'Global Reference List of 100 core indicators' in November 2014 (WHO 2014). Various countries and regions have also initiated consultative processes to define a core set of national and subnational mandatory and optional indicators, which also should show compatibility with global and regional initiatives. To be able to monitor this set of indicators, the HIS would first need to be able to access data from sources that traditionally have not been part of the HIS, and also to be linked with national and regional health observatories to enable effective dissemination, analysis, and use of information.

10.2.6 Health information systems challenges with health in the post-2015 development agenda

Many new health priorities are being included in the post-2015 (post-Millennium Development Goals) development agenda. These include the Sustainable Development Goals (SDGs), the Rio + 20 Open Working Group, and other UN Resolutions.

The Sustainable Development Goals has 17 goals and 169 targets. Though only the third SDG exclusively addresses public health, almost all the other goals directly or indirectly contribute to better health outcomes. A central narrative built into SDG-3, the health goal, is to maximize health for all ages with UHC as a means and an end in itself. These new priorities will require a reorientation of the HIS needed to support this post-2015 development agenda for health (United Nations Sustainable Development Summit 2015).

10.2.7 UN political declaration on prevention and control of non-communicable diseases

Adopted in 2011, this declaration requires setting up national targets and indicators measuring progress towards prevention and control of risk factors for non-communicable diseases (NCDs). Data on NCDs is often not integrated into the national HIS, making it difficult to use for advocacy, policy, and assessment of impact of interventions. A significant implication on HIS is to develop suitable indicators to monitor NCD programmes, and integrate with national HIS. Furthermore, there are various global surveys being done such as GATS (Global Adult Tobacco Survey) and GYTS (Global Youth Tobacco Survey) to monitor tobacco prevalence. These surveys (such as age categorizations) need to be harmonized with the data needed to generate the required indicators, and to be able to speak to the national HIS. Monitoring hypertension and blood sugar in individuals may require the need for biomarkers to also be incorporated into national HIS, representing novel challenges.

10.2.8 Complying with International Health Regulations (2005)

Building core capacities for disaster management and emergency preparedness involves strong HIS to support responses in disasters and emergencies, and to share information across the multiple parties involved. These HIS will require 'on demand' reporting periodicity, as contrasted with the monthly reporting which currently exists, and will also involve the use of mobile and handheld devices from areas of poor or destroyed infrastructure. This multiplicity of devices will raise key challenges of integration with national HIS.

10.2.9 Health systems strengthening in countries

Many elements of health system strengthening are captured in the WHO publication 'Everybody's business: strengthening health systems to improve health outcomes' (WHO 2007), which describes the six components of health systems, including HIS. In this understanding, a key aspect of health systems strengthening is enhancing the capacity of national HIS by improving reporting of births, deaths, causes of death, monitoring of exposure to risk factors, social determinants of health, morbidity, mortality and health system performance, and institutionalizing population-based surveys. In addition, HIS, with well-defined information flows, serves as a crucial ingredient of inter-sectoral coordination required across the board.

10.2.10 **Measurement and accountability**

This was a key outcome of a summit in Washington, 'Measurement and Accountability for Results in Health Summit' held from 9 to 11 June 2015, attended by major global health institutions (http://www.who.int/mediacentre/events/meetings/2015/measurement-accountability-health/en/). The focus on measurement and accountability will require the greater use of statistics and analytical features, which many of the current HIS are bereft of. Furthermore, skills for interpreting such indicators will also need to be developed.

Table 10.1 summarizes the implications of recent global health reforms on HIS.

Table 10.1 Implications of recent Global Health Initiatives on HIS

Health reform initiative	Implications on HIS
Universal health coverage	◆ Compiling and storing baseline data on coverage ◆ Need for name-based and encounter-based data ◆ HIS to cater to needs of different providers of financial coverage ◆ Indicators require data from non-HIS sources, raising the need for integration
Commission on Accountability for Women and Children	◆ Name-based and event-based tracking of women and child health related concerns (antenatal, delivery, immunization, etc.) ◆ Ability of name-based systems to be aggregated and linked with facility-based systems ◆ Ability to drill down from aggregate systems to individual names for better diagnosis and action
Strengthening of CRVS systems	◆ Strengthening systems of collecting data on births and deaths ◆ The HIS should speak to CRVS systems typically owned by Ministry of Justice or Interior ◆ Strengthening cause of death recording, based on ICD codes ◆ Integrating systems comprising CRVS such as notification, registration, verbal autopsy, generation of vital statistics, etc.
Accelerating EPI (Expanded Programme on Immunization)	◆ Stronger monitoring of individual immunization records through the development of immunization registries ◆ NHIS to have ability to identify dropout stages in the immunization life cycle, to better diagnose action ◆ Integrating information of cold chain equipment management with service coverage, to better manage demand and supply of vaccines

Health reform initiative	Implications on HIS
Monitoring core set of indicators	◆ Ensuring quality and timeliness of reporting of all data required for the generation of these core indicators ◆ Many of the data are coming from non-HIS sources, raising the need for integration of systems ◆ Standardization of nomenclature and reporting formats and frequencies within and across countries, ensure comparability across the reporting units ◆ Building strong skills to analyse, interpret data, and to take evidence-based action
Health in post-2015 development agenda— the Sustainable Development Goals.	◆ Many new and multidisciplinary priorities, requiring new types of data and indicators for monitoring ◆ To better monitor well-being at all stages of life, and of individuals' progress from the 'cradle to the grave'
UN political declaration on prevention and control of non-communicable diseases	◆ Integration of data of tobacco consumption coming from surveys with HIS ◆ Building capacities to process integrated data
Building core capacities for International Health Regulations	◆ Increasing focus on patient-level data requires stronger focus on privacy, security, confidentiality, etc. ◆ Stronger regulation in HIS will be required, as private players become more active with demands for insurance
Health systems strengthening in countries	◆ With more complexity, higher skills are needed in individuals to process, analyse, and use data ◆ Infrastructure requirements become more complex as the need to manage dependencies across systems increases ◆ Increasing amount of data needs to be collected from the community and non-health facility-based sources

Despite the strong informational content of these global health reform initiatives, their mutual links with HIS has rarely ever been explicitly cultivated, with some exceptions such as CoIA and EPI. In most LMICs, the existing architecture cannot be incrementally expanded to take in all these new demands, and thus requires a radical reconceptualization. We argue that, as both the nature of reforms and the HIS gain in complexity, it is imperative to explicitly design and develop their synergies.

10.3 Interdependence and Synergies: Health Sector Reform and Reform of National/Public Health Information Systems

The term 'health sector reform' denotes all 'sustained, purposeful change to improve the efficiency, equity and effectiveness of the health sector' (Berman

1995). We enunciate below ten normative aims to develop synergies between these and HIS strengthening efforts.

1. *The development of public health informatics is best where there is a clear stated national commitment to public health—where the government holds itself accountable for maintaining the health of populations—as different from being limited to providing access to those who seek healthcare.*

Expanded PHI necessarily works to integrate clinical individual-level information with the measurement of the health of populations. There is a stream of development of health informatics where the use of informatics for supporting individual patient-based clinical care has been emphasized, but little attention has been paid to measuring health outcomes and utilization at the population level. There is another stream of development of health informatics, in this instance more avowedly public health oriented, which measures only population health using aggregate numbers, but is limited to programme monitoring of vertical single disease control programmes. But these dichotomies are seen in health sector reform as well—where donors support single disease control programmes and selective health interventions, leaving the rest to market forces. In such contexts, the support for an Expanded PHI has historically been neglected.

Where there is commitment to Health for All and UHC, these concepts are interpreted to mean a comprehensive primary healthcare approach which is inclusive of most of the causes of illness and costs of care. Here then is a requirement for Expanded PHI. Though many developed nations achieved what would be now termed as UHC far before health informatics arrived, LMICs would find it essential to have the advantages of efficiency and effectiveness that digitization brings about to achieve such a universal outcome.

2. *Health information systems would be perceived and allowed to grow as dynamic systems, where health sector reforms are driven by an understanding of reimagining and shaping health systems as complex adaptive systems.*

Health sector reforms have been in the past perceived as a one-time effort to set in place institutions which will then allow market forces to act under the assumption it will lead to higher efficiencies. The paradigm is gradually changing; since as institutions and their requirements change, providing feedback through use, this leads to new requirements, unintended consequences, and new learning. Viewed through the lens of complex adaptive systems, policies and procedures often exist not because they are the most efficient, but because of high transaction costs shaped by path dependencies. 'Change often happens not when detailed plans are dictated from the top down, but when on the ground agents self-organise to maximise the equity and efficiency of health actions locally. When systems and organisations are complex, the greatest need is often the creation of an environment where locals can self-organise to develop innovative and context-appropriate approaches to health challenges through local organisations and networks' (Swanson *et al.* 2015). Again there is a synergy needed with a dynamic evolving HIS which supports and is supported by an evolving understanding of healthcare reform. Such an understanding is necessarily multidisciplinary, in the way we have defined Expanded PHI based on a 'systems approach'. Translated into the IT domain, it favours the building of open architectures (as contrasted to vertical and stand-alone systems not based on standards for interoperability with other systems), contextualization, and a plurality of methods for its development with action research at the core.

3. *Decentralization and participatory governance need an approach towards gathering and using information, which is embedded in an improved management culture.*

Health sector reforms are based on institutional theories and these emphasize the need for a movement towards governance that is more participatory and decentralized. Such a governance reform is best supported by an approach where meanings of 'what the data is telling us' are derived from 'conversations over data'. Systems that generate the necessary information are also best evolved if guided by a community of practice involving large numbers of groups with a high degree of interdisciplinarity collaboration. In Chapter 3, we discussed the problems involved in trying to promote a single version of the truth, and the role of power in this process. This is true not only about the management of information, but also about the management of health systems and reforms processes. A management culture that sees the workforce as creative collaborators rather than as unwilling, exclusively self-interested individuals who need to be controlled and commanded—or at best, aligned through incentives—is more willing to accept conversations over data as the way to promote the use of information, and communities of practice as the best way to develop HIS.

4. *Integration of IT into the work processes of the healthcare providers requires a reimagination and re-engineering of the work process itself, and brings several human resource policy implications.*

We discussed in Chapter 3 that as long as data entry remained one additional layer of work over the existing work processes and further, it is perceived to not bring in added value to the healthcare provider (the foundation of the national HIS), then the quality and use of information will forever remain limited. But integration of IT into the work process also needs a rethinking of the work processes and task allocations of the peripheral provider. If a provider in a hospital spends 90 seconds per patient then there is hardly any IT system that can solve the problem of quality of information or the quality of healthcare, which are intimately intertwined. Ad hoc solutions like adding an IT data entry operator at the level of the individual provider will never work for a number of reasons, including costs. If there is a time standard average of, say, 10 to 15 minutes per patient encounter, then the supporting IT system could be more effectively integrated with the existing work processes. In addition to efficiency improvements, the HIS should open up new possibilities for providing continuum of care across multiple visits and providers. This is the precise meaning of synergy—when the net output of the combination is more than the linear sum of the individual components.

5. *HIS reforms leading to an integration of multiple IT systems is a subset of the health sector reforms with the ambition of horizontal integration of vertical programmes.*

It is true that the chances of success and benefits of the former will depend on the pace and effectiveness of the latter. But it is also true that a push for integration of HIS can catalyse and accelerate the process of vertical programmes speaking to each other. With persistence of vertical programmes and their consequences for fragmentation, there are good reasons for a special focus on integration efforts of some programmes, with good capacities and resources in order to create models for success. These models could help explain resistance to integration, especially where the effort is a top-down push, insensitive to the way institutions function. More incremental bottom-up approaches do better, but that would mean a HIS that can manage such transitions and therefore actively promote it.

6. *Expanded PHI, rising as it were in LMICs from aggregate data for vertical programmes but now including name-based data, has to develop systems for privacy of data, data security, and ownership of data.*

These concerns of privacy, security, and ownership have been described in Chapter 5. In developed nations, there were already legal statutes that addressed these concerns with respect to medical records, which could then be adjusted to include electronic medical records. The first wave of health sector reforms in LMICs was not pressed to address these concerns, but now putting in place regulatory measures for legal and ethical issues related to name-based data should be a major concern. Expanded PHI, which calls for rolling individual data to create population-based data and 'drilling down' from population data to uncover the individual, needs to urgently address this issue. This requires urgent policy and regulation measures, and emerging HIS need to build compliance with them.

7. *Expanded PHI, as one form of big data, also needs to grapple with issues of the use of such information for research.*

Ethical concerns, especially as regards ownership of data, are present and so are epistemological concerns upon the meaning derived from such extended databases that big data involves. These concerns are areas that health sector reforms in LMICs remain blissfully unaware of, but such ignorance has its costs. There are potential threats to national sovereignty, and the bias, if not manipulation, of knowledge is what LMICs need to be cautious of. Establishing data science centres to guide research and practice are important priorities of policy reform efforts.

8. *Expanded PHI needs a considerable increase in organizational capacity but so does all of health sector reform.*

Most health sector reforms are best theorized as increases in organizational capacity. This involves the expansion of human resources, skills and infrastructure required for IT as simultaneously a means and an end for the increase of organizational capacity of healthcare systems. There are many key opportunities here for synergies, as alluded to in Chapter 5. Recapitulating, one important contribution is in supporting transitions in organization of healthcare delivery; another is in addressing the challenge of scale; a third is to ensure more effective surveillance of diseases, which in turn would enable decentralized planning and more responsive healthcare services; the fourth is a more sensitized engagement of development partners; and, finally a better informed and more effective governance framework.

9. *Institutional barriers for information and communications technology (ICT) introduction and use need institutional reform. And institutional reform requires skilled negotiation and astute and determined leadership—not easy conditions to meet. The introduction of ICT provides a context, in which the rules of the game—both formal and informal—that define the institutional relationships and work processes could be examined and re-worked.*

In Chapter 6, we discussed how existing institutions could be barriers to the introduction of ICTs and use of information. However, the introduction of reforms could also be perceived as an opportunity for addressing these very barriers, creating space and context for renegotiating the relationships. ICT introduction and health sector reforms justified by its introduction are facilitated if there are incentives for adopting the new system for all players, and not just the top management. And potentially, the willingness to examine the rules of the game can be used to redefine new rules in some key areas related to IT procurement; for example, to align rules made long back in entirely different contexts to the possibilities and complexities of modern technology access and use.

10. *The objectives of HIS systems are to improve performance of healthcare systems—but their own performance is a challenge. Common to both is the challenge of the governance of complex systems.*

One way of negotiating the complexity of governance requirements, discussed in some detail in Chapter 9, is the use of governance standards. The initial case studies of the use of governance standards are encouraging, and were these to be sustained, could not only be replicated in other nations, but also provide important clues to improving governance of healthcare systems. Important also is the learning that governance should take an inclusive perspective informed by social and political sciences and institutional theories, rather than one which is primarily technical. As discussed in Chapter 9, we also note that there are specific political choices to be made with respect to standards and the design of agencies responsible for setting up and implementing standards. These relate to the tension between the 'use values' of standards with respect to public health goals, and the 'exchange values' that relate to profits of IT industry. In health sector reform, there are also political choices to be made—usually related to how much emphasis is given to considerations of health equity; the ideological compulsions to include private providers and the terms of inclusion; how health needs are prioritized; and, how the needs of healthcare industry are negotiated. Quite often political choices are justified as if they are technical choices, making them suboptimal. Where governance is more participatory, and there is more representation for weaker and marginalized sections, or there are communities of practice within which technical alternatives can be worked out and presented, one could question—or at least ameliorate—suboptimal political choices. Thus, in Chapter 9 we highlighted why IT governance requires an enabling policy environment, which is consultative and supportive, constructive and creative, and does not hinder everyday work—but has clarity in regard to requirements. These requirements of good governance need to be expanded to cover the whole of health sector reform.

10.4 Moving Forward: At the Level of Policy, Academics, and Practice

The era when the health information systems could be perceived as a tool for health sector reforms is behind us. Health information systems,, in our understanding, are better perceived as co-evolving with health systems—requiring similar policy environments for facilitation and overcoming institutional barriers for their performance. However, this rather negative portrayal of the problems that beset current public health informatics should not in any way detract from the potential of ICTs to revolutionize the performance of healthcare systems in LMICs, or the determination to work towards this; as Gramsci once said, 'Pessimism of the intellect, optimism of the will'. It is the duty of academic thought to lay out the problems, barriers, and approaches, just as it is the task of implementers and governments to factor these in and move forward. The experience from other sectors, like banking and transport where informatics has revolutionized performance, provides the impetus to try again and do better.

An understanding of health sector reform which sees HIS as contributing to improved performance primarily through enhanced vertical accountability and results-based financing is a limited and questionable vision. Instead, enhancing organizational capacity with and through Expanded PHI needs to be made a central and guiding vision. Expanded PHI has the potential to transform the healthcare system to enable a dynamic learning and adapting system, to make decentralization effective, to improve quality of healthcare at costs that would be unimaginable for the developed world.

Clinical and biomedical informatics have already demonstrated that transformations are possible in individual patient care, in resource-rich Western environments. But with Expanded PHI, this continuity of care needs to be made possible across multiple episodes of care provision, providers, administrative levels, and sites of care. This approach has the potential to optimize solutions in contexts where there are massive structural constraints such as overcrowding, lack of skills, poor infrastructure, suboptimal healthcare-seeking behaviour, health inequities—all constraints that clinical informatics is seldom called on to grapple with. Finding appropriate solutions for Expanded PHI thus provides unique opportunities for innovations in both research and practice.

Currently existing HIS in LMICs have evolved to support roles of programme monitoring and measuring utilization of select services, including in a more limited way in logistics. Unfortunately, the last mile(s) of data quality and reliability, of use of information and the fragmentation of information, have remained stubbornly a bridge too far for the reform process. Expanded PHI holds out the promise of being able to close some of these gaps by identifying the barriers and overcoming them through a combination of technological and institutional innovation.

However, the real promise of Expanded PHI is in transforming the current models of care delivery, the measurement of health, and governance of health systems. But this requires informed political choices, including the build of a truly dynamic participatory information architecture by multiple communities of practice, where conversations over data interpret it, where legal and regulatory mechanisms safeguard the individual rights, and where systems of interoperability integrate and increase access to public information while helping to rationalize work burden of data providers. Such a choice has the potential to build the healthcare systems of the future, helping LMICs close the gap with developed nations in health outcomes at much lower cost and time requirements.

To reach out to this promise there are three levels of movement: policy; research and academia; and practice and activism. Each of these are now discussed.

10.4.1. Creating an enabling policy environment to guide health information systems development

Health policy has been defined by WHO (2015) as referring to 'decisions, plans, and actions that are undertaken to achieve specific healthcare goals within a society. An explicit health policy can achieve several things: it defines a vision for the future which in turn helps to establish targets and points of reference for the short and medium term. It outlines priorities and the expected roles of different groups; and it builds consensus and informs people' (http://www.who.int/topics/health_policy/en/).

So if expanding organizational capacity is the goal, what could be the specific objectives, targets, and points of reference with respect to public health informatics? What are the areas where sensitization is needed for policy and its content? Some areas of focus for policy development are now identified:

i)   *Standards:* Establish institutional processes for finalizing baseline standards, including relating to metadata for indicators, data sets, facilities, reporting periodicities, data exchange across systems and facilities, and creating an environment in which they can dynamically evolve. Important also is the need to create compliance mechanisms to these standards in the form of both incentives and disincentives.

ii) *Sourcing information:* Establishing legislation and systems to ensure reporting from all facilities, including the private sector, on a certain minimum mandatory information requirement regarding patterns of morbidity, mortality, and use of services. It also includes mandatory reporting of notifiable diseases from any source, reporting deaths with better cause-of-death reporting, and, wherever possible, medical certification of cause of death. Sourcing policies need to be supported with enabling dictionaries for data, indicators, and supporting practices. Furthermore, there needs to be clarity on what reporting is mandatory and what is optional, and to what level which data needs to be reported.

iii) *Integrating information:* This is a key policy requirement to address integration concerns which arise with the adoption and materialization of a data warehouse approach using a common set of tools. Other than standards and sources of information and dictionaries, this would also require: defining the nomenclature of organizational units and the linking hierarchy; establishing standards to exchange data across systems; presenting outputs and establishing data flows; and reporting practices of outputs. Frameworks like the Open Health Information Exchange have already provided architectural guidelines for this, but would need to be sensitively adapted to suit LMIC contexts.

iv) *Coordination:* Integration also requires actions at the institutional level, based on a positive policy environment created by governance mechanisms that are by design inter-sectoral; for example, to strengthen CRVS, and the innovative use of ICTs. Specific coordination mechanisms are needed between private and public sector healthcare providers, which span national, provincial, district, or city levels.

v) *Server-based administration:* While server-based systems make it technically easier to set up and support national HIS, there is a lot of policy support required to make things work. Policy guidelines need to detail the various server hosting options available, such as the cloud or in-house or third party data centres, and be able to provide explicit criteria to evaluate preferred options in particular contexts. Some of these criteria include:

   a. Adequate human capacity for server administration and operation, including for specific technologies in use for servers and database management.

   b. In the case of third party management—guidelines for building and managing procurement contracts.

   c. Reliable solutions for automated backups, including local off-server and remote backup.

   d. Stable connectivity and high network bandwidth for traffic to and from the server.

   e. Stable power supply, including a backup solution.

   f. Secure environment for the physical server including issues of access, theft, and fire.

   g. Presence of a disaster recovery plan, including a realistic strategy for ensuring effective service level agreements.

   h. Feasible, powerful, robust, and cost-effective hardware.

vi) *Procurements and Partnerships:* Establish systems of procurement that are appropriate to needs and agile enough to be able to respond to dynamic and changing environments. In most contexts, this is best assured by promoting an adherence to free and open source platforms, and standards and mechanisms that ensure interoperability of new systems. It also would imply a shift from procurement based on competitive bidding where each vendor works in a silo, to partnerships where development is collaborative and mutually reinforcing.

vii) *Accessing information and enabling data policy*: Data policy would need to define who will own the data, who would have access to it, who manages it, and how security and privacy would be ensured.

Data policy

Another set of policy measures relates to information access for public and all potential users, and one which would enable wider conversations including feedback around data not just limited to the government. The global Open Data movement is promoting free access and use of data and is gaining considerable momentum. See for example the Report from the 3rd International Open Data Conference 2015 in Ottawa for an overview (http://opendatacon.org/report/). India was an early adopter of the Open Data policy by legislating the Right to Infomration Act in 2005 (Government of India 2005) and the National Data Sharing and Accessibility Policy (NDSAP) in March 2012 (Government of India 2012), which was declaring a proactive disclosure of all non-sensitive data sets in open standards from ministries , departments, individual states, and from the public sector more generally. The https.data.gov.in Open Government Data Platform India portal was then created to publish these data sets. Here, anyone from anywhere can potentially access the portal and access, for example, an overview of the relevant Open Data and NDSAP-linked legislations (https://data.gov.in/catalogs/ministry_department/department-health-and-family-welfare). An unique feature of the Indian Open Data portal, directly linked to the right to information, is that users can request specific data sets and when 100 other users endorse the request, it becomes mandatory to release the data set (Parihar 2015). Technically, this Indian government portal illustrates how Open Data policy can be enabled through information portals with wide access, including to civil society.

Widening the scope and content of information dissemination

Information portals which enhance dissemination of information both within the health department and also to the public at large are going to be important to expand the role of public health informatics. Some key functions that a new generation of information portals could perform are to serve as an integrator of different data sources as it provides a single point of access to data of different types from different systems and databases, both dynamic and static. The portal can provide attractive and easy to use visualization tools to view data as maps, charts, reports, and tables in order to strengthen decision support. This allows providing value-added features to the information, such as geographical and thematic grouping, trends analysis, and linking with other useful websites. A portal can enable improving and widening the dissemination of health information by providing user-friendly interfaces to access and visualize data that do not require programmer-level intervention. Leveraging upon available new social media, interactivity of the portal can be strengthened, thus expanding the engagement of civil society.

Going back to the Indian Open Government portal and comparing with the above list of innovative new ways of presenting information, we see that it falls short on a number of the outlined issues; few of the data sets are provided with features of visualization and it is not easy to do comparions or analysis across data sets. The data sets are only uploaded to the portal and made available to the public and they are not prepared in a way that would enable analysis and comparisons across data sets. Isha Parihar asks 'How is open data changing India?' and notes that while data are made available in machine-readable format, a lot of editing and aggregation are needed in order to be able to make use of the data. 'Different departments collect and collate information in their respective silos using diverse formats and terminology, making it tough to use that data effectively' (Parihar 2015).

We can conclude that the need for standardization of meta data and terminologies discussed in this book in relation to HIS are as valid in the area of Open Data and the publication of data from accross departments using portal technology. Furthermore, big data can only be made useful for LMICs, if it has these characteristics of open data.

Human resources policies and capacity development

Materializing Expanded PHI needs a new breed of HR professional. To build this, policy support is required in many areas such as curriculum, institutions, testing, and certification. These need to cover a wider spectrum of skill sets including IT, statistics, big data analytics, and various others. Some specific measures in this regard include:

i) Curriculum redesign in colleges of medicine, community health, and in nursing schools to include modules in public health informatics. Help create formal collaboration between informatics and public health departments and schools and universities to have more comprehensive courses in public health informatics.

ii) Improve and standardize in-service training courses for different cadres of health staff.

iii) Support the development of Master's programmes on public health informatics as an institutional base for wider educational programmes.

iv) Help establish centres and networks of excellence in areas of cutting-edge knowledge areas such as big data analytics, which could:

a. Promote the use of best practice design approaches, such as web-based data warehousing and 'cloud' server hosting.

b. Provide technical and capacity support to units in the design, development, and implementation of software systems and processes.

c. Promote the use of standard open source software in line with global best practices.

d. Create and disseminate technical resources such as standards, user manuals, software use guides, and other resources.

e. Identify other institutions, such as universities and research centres, to provide technical capacities to their students customized to the country's requirements.

f. Help create mechanisms for mutual knowledge transfer across and within countries.

10.4.2 Implications for research and academia: Establishing theoretical foundations for Expanded PHI

Another frontier of advancement for Expanded PHI is in the generation of new knowledge. This calls for examination of the academic environment, in which HIS is taught and in which research is conducted. Currently public health informatics is classified within universities as an academic subdiscipline within the computer science and information technology department, or within the library and information sciences department, or within schools of public health. As discussed in Chapter 1, research in this domain is largely non-existent in LMICs, with nearly no place where knowledge is treated with a multidisciplinary perspective.

Formulating research challenges around Expanded PHI

The design, development, implementation and evolution of HIS for Expanded PHI will be fraught with multiple challenges, and these can be categorized under three broad research domains: use of information; choice of technology and innovation; and institutions of governance. These are now discussed.

Use of information We shall discuss some of the areas where use of information needs to contribute.

How can HIS contribute to priority setting and measurement of progress towards realizing health sector reforms/health systems strengthening? Health systems strengthening requires an understanding of which diseases are more prevalent, and their contribution to the burden of disease and out of pocket expenditure. This raises challenges relating to measurement of coverage, utilization of different healthcare services, and out of pocket expenditure on different drugs. There will be different gaps in institutional capacity to take action based on the reform priorities identified. The ability to generate more information will change the way in which progress is measured and raise new demands for information.

How can HIS support health equity measures towards UHC? This requires an understanding of the criteria for identifying exclusion and marginalization in relation to services and population subgroups. There are ongoing challenges of designing and interlinking equity measures to guide resource allocation. Measuring population coverage to understand social exclusion, barriers to access, and greater financial risk and hardship are areas where research is urgently required.

How can HIS add value at all levels of the health hierarchy? This requires an understanding of informational needs for primary care providers, mid-level managers, and policy makers. Designing appropriate ICTs to provide appropriate value—at every level of use, as different from only for the top—is a key challenge, along with building the users' capacity to make effective use of these ICTs.

How do divergent interests, including conflicts, operate around information? How is it negotiated in a constructive manner? This requires understanding both the explicit and the implicit programme theories of different stakeholders—how they perceive information as leading to change—and what the availability of information does to existing power relationships. Are there benefits to some for certain types of information to be suppressed or falsified, and can information empower weaker stakeholders to make more informed choices?

Choice of technology and innovation

What are the ecosystemic determinants of innovation and technology choice in development of HIS? This requires an understanding of the different stakeholders and their influences on technology choices. It depends on the ability of the ecosystem to consider available alternatives, and of the infrastructural conditions involved in shaping technological choices. It relates to the political economy of information and of IT—who sources the information; how is it produced, distributed, consumed, and paid for; who profits from it; and how are these different interests represented (or not) in the structures of governance and technology choices.

What are appropriate design strategies for low-cost and frugal innovation-based applications? This requires an understanding of how social, technical, and institutional conditions can shape choices for developing frugal innovation. Innovation efforts that focus primarily on technologies are not likely to succeed, but also need to be accompanied with social and institutional innovations. Frugal innovation will most effectively materialize only at the intersections of technical, institutional, and social innovation (Bhatti 2012).

What are appropriate strategies for integration and interoperability? This requires an understanding of how historical existing systems and data can be effectively integrated with the new; and the technical and institutional strategies required to enable them. Modern ICT solutions, indeed provide the potential to address these challenges, but they need to be accompanied with a deep understanding of the question of 'why' integration is required. Long periods of time are required to allow such efforts to come to fruition, as these are not just technical questions, but require the renegotiation of historically embedded institutions.

What are the appropriate strategies for technology assessment and evaluation of information systems? In areas of growing technological complexity and contestation, what institutional arrangements and processes would help optimal choices to be made? How are value-for-money propositions with respect to ICT assessed? How do we measure the effectiveness of the contribution that HIS makes to improved health sector performance when it itself is the tool of measurement, and when so many factors are at work in parallel?

Institutions of governance

What appropriate hybrids of centralization and decentralization are required? This requires understanding existing models of centralization and decentralization of the healthcare systems, and how these shape trajectories for the new systems, including the supporting HIS. The challenge is to design appropriate hybrid models that are appropriately contextualized. Large technology initiatives tend to bring with them top-down approaches following grand plans, but these are more often than not prone to failure. While a guiding vision is indeed important, these need to be informed by practices on the ground. Building such hybrid models is a non-trivial challenge, and needs to be actively governed through research and practice.

What is the regulatory environment required to secure privacy of information? This requires an understanding of the existing regulatory environment and gaps therein with respect to health sector reforms and the demands of new ICTs. A design challenge is to develop appropriate incentives and sanctions for private sector providers with respect to data, and to answer the related question of 'who should own personal data'? Simultaneously, the public needs to be made aware of their rights on information pertaining to their health, and the means to try and ensure them.

What are the appropriate decision-making structures required around technology? This requires an understanding of the existing decision-making models around health system issues, and how these can be modified and made more responsive to local priorities within frameworks of contemporary health reforms. This will necessarily require multisectoral models for HIS governance, which by definition are difficult to establish.

Exploring these research questions would need to be guided by novel theoretical and empirical approaches, which we now discuss.

Guiding theoretical approaches The guiding theoretical approaches need to be multidisciplinary, drawing from the domains of informatics, public health, science and technology studies, and development. Some specific approaches are discussed.

From science and technology studies (Latour 1999), we learn that 'airplanes don't fly, but airlines do', implying that technology on its own cannot achieve much, but requires the alignment of socio-technical heterogeneous networks including institutions, culturally situated work practices, technical systems, infrastructure, and many others. A direct implication for Expanded PHI is the nature of networks that are required, and how can they be enabled and evolved in specific contexts. Theories of information infrastructure from the informatics domain (Monteiro and Hanseth 1996; Ciborra and Hanseth 1998; Hanseth and Lytinen 2010) provide multiple supporting concepts on how to approach such network building. For example, they emphasize the role of history in terms of the 'installed base', and how strategies of cultivation need to sensitively leverage on what already exists while shaping the new. This contrasts with the oft-repeated approach of trying to build systems by starting on a clean slate.

Informatics and organization studies have articulated various models of decision-making, critiquing rationalistic approaches, which can provide insights to the problematic of use of information which is of central concern in Expanded PHI. While information is a necessary condition to ensure action, it is by no means sufficient (Latifov 2013) requiring many other pieces to be put in place. Kelly *et al.* (2013) emphasize the approach of 'conversations around data' between different stakeholder groups to trigger action and build a supporting information culture, rather than adopting rational models of decision-making.

While informatics research has focused extensively on building innovations, there is more limited research done on how technology choices are made. However, some guiding design principles can be noteworthy to guide such choices. For example—how do new choices account for the installed base, and can leverage on the positives that exist, as contrasted with adopting clean slate approaches (Aansted 2002). Another implication concerns the need to balance the needs of the global with locally situated circumstances, so that systems are locally specific, while also allowing easy generalization to other contexts (Rolland and Monteiro 2002). New technologies should support 'flexible standards' (Braa and Sahay 2012), where the local user is given autonomy, but within a metalevel framework which all players need to follow to ensure compliance to standards. Research into participatory design methods, a foundational aspect of informatics research, can provide useful inputs on how technology choices should be made. Research into the scalability (Sahay and Walsham 2006) and sustainability (Braa *et al.* 2004) of systems provides important criteria to consider in making new technology choices. Given the extremely resource-constrained environments in which new technologies are introduced, they must necessarily be guided by cost-effectiveness and 'frugal innovation' criteria (Bhatti 2012).

Governance concerns the institutional structure within which decisions around Expanded PHI are made (Sahay *et al.* 2014). Traditional institutions are historically and socially embedded and thus difficult to change (Latifov and Sahay 2012), and respond to the multisectoral and flexible structures required for Expanded PHI. Policies made at the top without hearing the voice of lower levels are bound to fail because of the limited overlap between formal institutions and informal constraints existing at the local sites of interventions (Piotti *et al.* 2006). Findings from neo-institutional theory can inform about the stability of institutions, and within this the challenge of change, through highlighting the contradictions between the old and the new (Nicholson and Sahay 2009). Strategies around deinstitutionalization (Nicholson and Sahay 2009) and institutional entrepreneurship (Hardy and Maguire 2008) can help design appropriate governance models in new institutions.

While these different conceptual inputs to design and to development dimensions are paramount, insights from development theorists like Sen (1999) urge us to look at the developmental impacts, such as 'does the HIS enable individuals to pursue the healthcare choices they value?', and the question posed by Walsham (2012) 'are ICTs contributing to build a better world'? (Walsham 2012).

Guiding methodological approaches The adopted methodologies should seek to address research questions such as: What are the different information use cases for multiple stakeholder groups that Expanded PHI needs to support?; How can information requirements for these systems be understood based on appropriately contextualized participatory design techniques?; How can prototyping methods be used to develop HIS which are flexible, locally relevant, and able to evolve with emerging needs?; What are the appropriate governance models for these systems to best support aims of financial inclusion and poverty reduction in accessing healthcare?; and—What are the socio-technical implementation challenges and appropriate strategies needed to address them?

The required methodologies would typically involve combinations of action research, realist evaluation, and comparative case study frameworks with action research at the core. A key principle underlying action research is that we learn better in collectives than as single units, and for this networks of action (Braa *et al.* 2004) need to be enabled at global and country levels comprising of university departments, Ministries of Health, policymaking bodies, technology providers, and civil society organizations. Action research can help generate theoretical and practical knowledge on how collaborating nodes in the network can be made self-organizing and self-sustaining, contributing to increased learning. Interpretive approaches (Walsham 1993) would be useful in understanding the different stakeholders' perspectives towards Expanded PHI, and how inter-subjectivity can be achieved.

Realist evaluation methods (Pawson and Tilley 1997) are especially relevant for informing management choices and designing scaled-up strategies. It represents a new form of strategic thinking and critical analysis of public managers' action with respect to decision-making (Barzeley 2001), and to help identify 'what works in which circumstances and for whom'? rather than merely 'does it work'? This perspective helps to analyse the underlying generative mechanisms that explain 'how' the outcomes were caused and the influence of context. This approach can help to understand how interventions have implicit programme theories that specify how a set of mechanisms generate key outcomes; intended as well as unintended. This approach helps to analyse particular situations and the kind of knowledge that is entailed, with a specific emphasis on the participation of individuals and how they contribute or not to the success of the programme, as contrasting with adopting scientific experimental methods which seek to be objective and value and context-neutral.

Methodologically, comparative case study analysis with a longitudinal design can help to develop unique research insights across countries, districts, or provinces currently engaged in developing Expanded PHI. Mixed methods of data collection would be required; including secondary data analysis, interviews, observation, participatory design, software prototyping, and realist implementation evaluation. While secondary data analysis will help to understand the contextual conditions of Expanded PHI models, interviews and observations can provide insights to informational priorities of stakeholder groups, existing flows and gaps of information, and challenges of managing the transition to the new HIS. Participatory design techniques, appropriately contextualized, can help to ensure appropriate needs and local knowledge are included as essential inputs into prototyping methods and in evolving the HIS. Data analysis can involve inductively developing research themes from the data for each case; generating cross-theme analyses across the cases; and developing broader theoretical inferences around the themes of use of information, technology choice and innovation, and governance of HIS.

10.4.3 **Establishing communities of practice and activist networks**

This understanding of Expanded PHI has relevance not only for policy makers and academics, but also for practitioners and activists who seek to shape the development of health informatics as a contributor to a more democratic and equitable vision of healthcare systems.

The development of this field of public health informatics has historically been supported by the contribution of communities of practice, such as related to open source software development. Increasingly, in recent times organizations have become more conscious of this contribution, and have tried to enable planned action networks and well-financed and planned communities of practice. The growth of social media has also contributed to mobilizing these networks, and in realizing their potential to shape policy and also design better working solutions on the ground. Action needs to thus enable seamless and permeable inter-institutional spaces where IT developers, information users, public health experts, and academics meet informally and exchange ideas and learn from one another. Similar learning processes and environments need to be enabled at the policy level—where development financing agencies, technical assistance teams linked to donors, and national policy makers can interact with the problem-solving and implementing teams on the ground—so that they are more informed of the existence and possible solutions for the 'wicked' problems of this domain.

10.5 **Conclusion**

Health informatics is a young discipline which has seen an explosive growth in the last two decades, and within this, a newer and even younger discipline—public health informatics—is being shaped. Even as this book goes to print, a large multitude of universities globally are beginning to offer postgraduate courses and doctoral programmes in public health informatics, text books are being written, new journals are starting, new divisions, and even new companies starting up are growing exponentially. However, there is already a need to reflect on and rethink the scope of this discipline and the possible directions its development could take. Whereas public health informatics may have emerged in parallel to clinical informatics, or even as a subdiscipline within health informatics, in this notion of Expanded PHI that we tentatively advance—PHI is the overarching architecture—and other dimensions like electronic medical records or clinical informatics become its subsets. But for this to be globally accepted, the rethinking of public health informatics would have to span policy, research, and practice.

This book is a small but important step in this direction—our modest contribution towards nudging the development of this discipline in such a direction.

10.6 **References**

Aansted, M. (2002) Cultivating Networks: Implementing Surgical Telemedicine, Ph. D thesis, University of Oslo, Norway.

Barzeley, M. (2001). *The New Public Management* (1st edition). University of California Press, Berkeley, CA.

Berman, P. (1995). *Health Sector Reform in Developing Countries: Making Health Development Sustainable.* Harvard University Press, Boston, MA.

Bhatti, Y.A. (2012). What is frugal, what is innovation? Towards a theory of frugal innovation. Available at: http://ssrn.com/abstract=2005910 or http://dx.doi.org/10.2139/ssrn.2005910

Braa, J. and **Sahay, S.** (2012). Participatory design within the HISP network. *Routledge International Handbook of Participatory Design.* Routledge, Oxford, UK, pp. 235.

Braa, J., Monteiro, E., and **Sahay, S.** (2004). Networks of action: sustainable health information systems across developing countries. *Mis Quarterly,* **23**(3), 337–62.

Ciborra, C.U. and **Hanseth, O.** (1998). From tool to Gestell agendas for managing the information infrastructure. *Information Technology & People,* **11**(4), 305–27.

Commission on Information and Accountability for Women's and Children's Health (2012). Accountability for Women's and Children's Health, WHO [Online]. Available at: http://www.who.int/woman_child_accountability/about/coia/en/index5.html [Last accessed 14 October 2015].

Government of India (2005). *Right to Information Act, 2005,* Ministry of Law and Justice, Government of India.

Government of India (2012). National Data Sharing and Accessibility Policy-2012 (NDSAP-2012). Department of Science and Technology, Government of India.

Hanseth, O. and **Lyytinen, K.** (2010). Design theory for dynamic complexity in information infrastructures: the case of building internet. *Journal of Information Technology,* **25**(1), 1–19.

Hardy, C. and **Maguire, S.** (2008). Institutional entrepreneurship. In: **Greenwood, R., Oliver, C., Suddaby, R.,** and **Sahlin, K.** (eds.). *The Sage Handbook of Organizational Institutionalism.* Sage Publications, Thousand Oaks, CA, pp. 198–217.

Kelly, S., Noonan, C., and **Sahay, S..** (2013). Re-framing evidence-based public health: from Scientific decision-making to occasioning conversations that matter. Proceedings of the 12th International Conference on Social Implications of Computers in Developing Countries, Ocho Rios, Jamaica.

Latifov, M.A. and **Sahay, S.** (2012). Data warehouse approach to strengthen actionability of health information systems: Experiences from Tajikistan. *The Electronic Journal of Information Systems in Developing Countries,* **53**(1), 53.

Latifov, M.A (2013). Global Standards and Local Health Information System Applications: Understanding their interplay in the context of Tajikistan (Doctoral thesis). Department of Informatics, University of Oslo, Norway.

Latour, B. (1999). *Pandora's Hope: On the Reality of Science Studies*. Harvard University Press, Cambridge, MA.

Monteiro, E., and Hanseth, O. (1996). Social shaping of information infrastructure: on being specific about technology. In: Orlikowski, W.J., Walsham, G., Jones, R., and De Gross, J.I. (eds.). *Information Technology and Changes in Organizational Work*. Chapman & Hall, London, UK, pp. 325–43.

Nicholson, B. and Sahay, S. (2009). Deinstitutionalization in the context of software exports policymaking in Costa Rica. *Journal of Information Technology*, 24(4), 332–42.

Parihar, I. (2015) How is Open Data Changing India. Available at: https://www.weforum.org/agenda/2015/02/how-is-open-data-changing-india/

Pawson, R., and Tilley, N. (1997). *Realistic Evaluation*. Sage Publications, Thousand Oaks, CA.

Piotti, B., Chilundo, B., and Sahay, S. (2006). An institutional perspective on health sector reforms and the process of reframing health information systems: Case study from Mozambique. *The Journal of Applied Behavioral Science*, 42(1), 91–109.

Rolland, K.H. and Monteiro, E. (2002). Balancing the local and the global in infrastructural information systems. *The Information Society*, 18(2), 87–100.

Sahay, S. and Walsham, G. (2006). Scaling of health information systems in India: challenges and approaches. *Information Technology for Development*, 12(3), 185–200.

Sahay, S., Sundararaman, T., and Mukherjee, M (2014), Building locally relevant models for Universal Health Coverage and its implications for Health Information Systems: Some Reflections from India. HELINA, Accra, Ghana, October 2014.

Sen, A. (1999). *Development as Freedom*. Oxford University Press, Oxford, UK.

Swanson, R. C., Atun, R., Best, A., *et al.* (2015). Strengthening health systems in low-income countries by enhancing organizational capacities and improving institutions. *Globalization and Health*, 11(1), 5. https://globalizationandhealth.biomedcentral.com/articles/10.1186/s12992-015-0090-3

The Partnership for Maternal, Newborn and Child Health (2013). PMNCH Knowledge Summary #27 Death reviews: maternal, perinatal and child. [Online]. Available at: http://www.who.int/pmnch/knowledge/publications/summaries/ks27/en/ [Last accessed 14 October 2015].

United Nations (2011). Sixty-sixth session Agenda item 117—Political Declaration of the High-level Meeting of the General Assembly on the Prevention and Control of Non-communicable Diseases—A/66/L.1 [Online]. Available at: http://www.who.int/nmh/events/un_ncd_summit2011/political_declaration_en.pdf?ua=1 [Last accessed 14 October 2015]

//www.un.org/en/ga/info/draft/index.shtml&Lang=E [Last accessed 14 October 2015].

United Nations (2015). Sustainable Development Summit 2015 25–27 September 2015, New York. Available at: https://sustainabledevelopment.un.org/post2015/summit (Last accessed: 19 July 2016).

Walsham, G. (1993) *Interpreting Information Systems in Organizations*. Wiley, Chichester, UK

Walsham, G. (2012). Are we making a better world with ICTs? Reflections on a future agenda for the IS field. *Journal of Information Technology*, 27(2), 87–93.

WHO (2007). Everybody's business—strengthening health systems to improve health outcomes: WHO's framework for action. [Online]. Available at: http://www.who.int/healthsystems/strategy/everybodys_business.pdf

WHO (2012). The work of WHO in the Eastern Mediterranean Region: Annual report of the Regional Director 1 January–31 December 2012. [Online]. Available at: http://www.emro.who.int/annual-report/2012/index.html

WHO (2014). Global Reference List of 100 Core Indicators: Working Paper 5 [Online]. Available at: http://www.who.int/healthinfo/country_monitoring_evaluation/GlobalRefListCoreIndicators_V5_17Nov2014_WithoutAnnexes.pdf [Last accessed 14 October 2015].

WHO (2015). Health policy [Online]. Available at: http://www.who.int/topics/health_policy/en/ [Last accessed 14 October 2015].

Index